FINDING PURPOSE

after

SEXUAL ABUSE AND TRAUMA

Living Beyond
Pain and Finding
My True Identity in God

JUANITA R. WILLIAMS

Table of Contents

Introduction

This journey is not for the faint of heart. It takes courage, perseverance, trust, and hope in God, our creator. Tearing down the old me piece by piece is not easy, but I have to press forward. Before starting this journey, I was unaware of how much I was slowly deteriorating. My wounded soul needed healing, and my spirit desperately needed reviving. Through this journey, I discovered life beyond the existence of pain and my true identity in God.

Life is a lesson. My journey was filled with a lot of twists, turns, speed bumps, and potholes. I even experienced some wind storms, tornados, and earthquakes, but God kept me through them all. Navigation is key. From youth to maturity, we are finding our place, our pace, and ourselves. Some journeys are pleasant; some are not. What is most important is what you learn from it.

I've learned some great things on my journey, like how to cook and clean. How to comb my hair, the jury is still out on that one. How to ride a bike, drive a car and even how to check the oil and fill the radiator. I also learned how to be a mother and wife, which is not easy but rewarding.

There are some other things I learned on this journey that was not so great. I learned how to lie and hide. I learned that if someone, because for their selfishness, wants to take something from you, they can and will, and you will pay the consequences. I learned that the people that say they care about and love you don't always mean it.

I also learned about sex, masturbation, and pornography at a young age. As you will learn in the chapters that follow, my first experience with sex was as a preteen when I was sexually violated.

On my journey, there are things I experienced from adolescence to adulthood that broke me to my core. I was abandoned, bullied, and shunned. Ostracized and marginalized. Those things caused me great pain. What broke me was the molestation and rape. I never asked for this to happen to me. Nobody does. I never asked why it happened. Life happens, whether good or bad. God is not surprised. I still don't quite understand it all, but I have since come to realize that all things work together for my good and God's glory. *I don't mean to say that I have already achieved these things or that I have already reached perfection. But I press on to possess that perfection for which Christ Jesus first possessed me. No, dear brothers and sisters, I have not achieved it, but I focus on this one thing: Forgetting the past and looking forward to what lies ahead, I press on to reach the end of the race and receive the heavenly prize for which God, through Christ Jesus, is calling us. (Philippians 3: 12-14 NLT)*

In 2016, God reminded me while watching a sermon by Pastor Sarah Jakes-Roberts, of what He called me to do. In 1996 God called me to preach His word. Although I knew He called me years ago, I was not operating in that calling because I did not have a full understanding of the call. I thought Him calling me to preach meant I needed to stand on a platform behind the sacred desk and proclaim His word.

At my current place of worship, women are not allowed to preach. Because my husband said, this is where the Lord led him, I trusted his lead and followed him. To be honest, because I was not allowed to operate in my calling, I was a little frustrated. I questioned if the Lord led my husband, or was it his choice.

Because women are not allowed to preach, I came up with my own plan. I never gave up on my calling. I was determined to be obedient to God. I decided to modify my calling. I made up in my mind that I would proclaim God's word through song. After a few years of wrestling within myself about my calling, I resolved not to be concerned about the preaching part but focus on ministering through song. I laugh at myself while writing this because God did not ask for my help. In 2016 after getting the reminder about my calling, I took a series of steps to walk in my calling. I talked to my leaders and my Pastor. Still to no avail but I pressed on. I was determined to be obedient to God regardless of what man said.

God reminded me of a conversation I had with a First Lady a few years back. During that conversation, she explained what the word preach meant. To proclaim the word of God. She also explained that I could proclaim His word anywhere. It didn't necessarily have to be on a platform behind the sacred desk. When she initially told me that, I didn't quite get it. My understanding was, when you are called, you stand in the pulpit and preach. Thank God for enlightenment. The platform the Lord gives is not necessarily inside four walls. It can be anywhere. On a street corner, at the grocery store, at your place of employment, provided it's not prohibited. But even if it is, our lives are a sermon. We don't have to say a word, but we must live according to the word of God.

Our life experiences can preach, and our testimonies can bring healing, hope, and wholeness. *Give thanks to the Lord, for He is good! His faithful love endures forever. Has the Lord redeemed you? Then speak out! (Psalm 107:1-2 NLT)*

In 2018 I purchased the book Wholeness by Best Selling Author Pastor Toure' Roberts. I started reading it but had to put it down. I was flooded with memories from my childhood that were very painful. I could only read the book in small doses. The more I read, the more I began to understand the tests and trials I experienced in life. I realized that although I had been set free many years ago, I was still operating in brokenness.

In the following chapters, you will read my story. This is not an autobiography, but a testimony of the struggles and challenges I faced, the effect they had on my life and my journey to healing, freedom, and wholeness. There were a lot of difficulties that I didn't quite understand, but God was with me through them all. Will you join me as I begin my Journey to Wholeness?

CHAPTER 1

Beginnings

Looking for perfection in imperfect people will keep you on
a mental and emotional rollercoaster forever. You have
to find that inner peace hidden deep in the crevices
of your mind, heart, and spirit for yourself while walking in
the realization that you'll never find perfection in your he-
roes. Have they failed you? Or have you failed them?
Create your own footsteps instead of trudging through the
deep, muddy footsteps of others. Your footsteps may lead
to the same destination. You just had to create a different
path to reach it.
Benjamin Lamar Thornton

I found an article on the internet written by Melissa
Mayntz titled Definition of a Blended Family. It states
the simple definition of a blended family, also called a
stepfamily, reconstituted family, or a complex family, is a
family unit where one or both parents have children from a
previous relationship, but they have combined to form a new
family. The parents may or may not then have children with
each other. Traditionally, the parents of a blended family
would be married, often after divorce or death of a previous

spouse. But modern blended families may have married parents or cohabitant parents, both can serve as role models for the children without a marriage ceremony.

My mother and father had seven children: six sons and one daughter. My father used to tell his testimony of how he and my mother prayed for a daughter. I am the result of their prayer. I was their last child. Unfortunately, my mother's time with me was cut short. The Saturday after Thanksgiving in 1967, she got out of bed but never returned. That night she went home to be with the Lord.

The only vivid memory I have of my mother was that fateful night in 1967. Unfortunately, I don't remember all of the details. After talking with my oldest brother about that night, he filled in the rest of the details.

My mother got out of bed and went into the bathroom. She called out for my second oldest brother, who did not hear her. My oldest brother got up to see what she needed. He saw her holding on to the sink. He said she pointed towards to toilet. He tried to help her sit down, but she fell instead and hit her head on the bathtub. She was too heavy for him to hold up. At some point, my second oldest brother got out of bed and tried to help her get up, but neither of them could lift her.

When I came out of the bedroom, I saw her laying on the bathroom floor. I did not know what to do. I do not know long she was there. My oldest brother told me my Dad came home, pulled my mother out of the bathroom, and laid her in the hallway. My father then told my brother to go to a neighbor's and call the ambulance. I don't remember seeing any of those details.

Finally, I saw my Dad coming up the stairs, followed by two men in green uniforms. They were carrying a stretcher.

After they put my mother on the gurney, my Dad told me she reached out and grabbed my hand as they were taking her down the stairs. Another detail about that night I do not remember. Because I only have vague memories of my mother, I am forever grateful my Dad shared that with me.

My Dad was determined to keep his children together, so he raised us by his self for three years. He got married again in 1971 to my step-mother who had six children of her own. After they were married life for me would never be the same.

As a child, even though I didn't have my mother anymore, I remember being happy and free. I remember waking up without a care in the world. Life as I knew it was great. It was my Dad, my brothers and me.

My Dad had quite a few awesome people who he trusted to help take care of his crew. I remember one sunny Saturday morning a family friend combed my hair. Back then, I had a head full of very thick, long hair. The family friend decided to let me wear my hair in an afro. Feeling the wind blow through my hair and the sun shining on my face was exhilarating. I was happy and free.

I loved riding my bike and going to the Big Field (an area in the Taft Homes with a basketball court and a playground) which was just a short walk from our apartment. I was always accompanied by one of my brothers or one of our family friends. I also loved going outside to play with the kids in the neighborhood.

There was a little girl who used to come to our apartment just about every day to play with me. We ran up, and down the sidewalk, I could not go very far, or we played in the dirt just outside my back door. We had fun for hours; then our playtime would turn sour. It never failed. Every time she came to play with me, we would end up in an argument.

She would then stand up and say the words that to this day, will get you a beat down. Those words you should never say in any circumstance are "Yo Mama."

Why did she have to go there? Every time. I do not remember what our silly arguments were about, but without fail, she would say those offensive words. When she uttered those words, I would chase her down to the end of the block. I was not allowed to cross the street. When she got across the street, she would stick her tongue out and run home.

Every time she came back to my apartment to play, she would apologize. I would accept her apology; we would play, argue, then she would repeat those words.

One day the little girl came over to play like she usually did. We played together for a while, argued, then she repeated those words. She ran, I chased her, she crossed the street, stuck her tongue out, and ran home. But this time, my brother was standing at the back door and heard her utter those infamous words. He called me in the house and told me the next time the girl comes to play with me, to invite her into the apartment. He devised a plan. Once she was inside, we would trap her in the utility closet. I would then threaten her for saying those horrible words, then beat her up.

The little girl did not come back for a few days. When she finally came over to play, I invited her into the house then operation utility closet beat down began. I threatened her and pushed her into the utility closet. My brother and family friend blocked the doorway so she could not escape. My brother handed me a belt. I proceeded to threaten her, push her, and threaten her with the belt. We finally let her out of the utility closet. She ran to the back door and without fail, repeated those offensive words. I hardly saw her after that incident and she never came back to play with me again.

One Saturday morning, after getting out of bed, I was told my brother ran away again. I was too young to really understand what that meant, but I knew one of my brothers was not in the apartment. From what I recall, my Dad was not at the house either. When he returned, we all piled into his Electric 225 Buick and went searching for my brother. We rode around for a while, then rode down to the riverfront. We found my brother sitting on a bench facing the river. My Dad got out the car, walked up to my brother, snatched him off the bench, and took him home. My brother had run away before, and it wouldn't be the last time he would run away.

Dad ran a tight ship. Every Saturday, as I remember, was cleaning day. We were all given chores and were expected to complete them. Bedtime for everyone was 8:00 p.m., no compromising. Although my Dad was strict, we had fun family time as well.

My father married again when I was 6-years-old. The woman he married had six children from a previous marriage, three girls and three boys.

After my father married again, we moved from the Taft Homes to a house on Third and Webster. It was a large house with several bedrooms, a large kitchen, and a large basement. With 13 children, it was needed. Blending two families wasn't easy. It felt like we were just thrown together and expected to live as one big happy family. That didn't happen. We argued and fought. Sometimes there were individual fights; other times, it was one family against the other family. Most of this happened when both parents were gone.

During those family battles, I would be surrounded by my brothers. I always felt protected. After the arguments were over, my brothers would go upstairs to their rooms, and

I would be left by myself. My protection, my covering was gone. My happy, free life was not so happy and free anymore.

One night after one of those quarrels, everyone scattered to various rooms in the house. Before I could leave the hallway, where the dispute happened, a person I will refer to as Ina threatened me.

When our parents finally arrived home, it was close to bedtime. I tried to stay in the living room as long as I could. I was afraid of what might happen. I made small talk with my step-mother and asked random questions. I stalled as long as I could until she made me go to bed.

I slowly got up from the chair I was sitting in. The bedroom I shared with the girls was on the first floor. I walked unhurriedly down the hallway. I stood at the door for a minute; my heart was racing. I gently turned the doorknob and opened the door gradually. The room was dark and quiet. I felt a sense of relief. I tiptoed into the room so as not to wake anyone and closed the door softly behind me. I thought everyone was asleep. My bed was on the other side of the room. To get to my bed, I had to walk past the bed where Ina slept. As soon as I started walking towards my bed, Ina threatened again. My happy, free life was gone.

Soon after that, the bullying and shunning began. On any given day, I would get threatened or shunned. I guess that's when I became a conformer, to be obedient or compliant. I don't like chaos or confusion, so to keep the peace, I would comply or avoid.

I saw and experienced a lot while living in the house on Third and Webster. I was outside playing in the yard one day when I saw three teenage girls jump on another girl close in age. They punched, knocked her to the ground, and kicked her. Somehow her head ended up under a car. When the fight was finished, the girls walked away, leaving the other girl laying on the ground. When the victim stood up, I saw a large gash over her left eye. I was frightened. I stood up and starting walking towards our house all the while looking at the victim. By the time I reached the steps, she was right behind me. I walked up to the stairs and onto the porch. I opened the screen door, and she walked in as I held the door. She sat down in the chair, and I went to get my step-mother. My step-mother helped her and allowed her to make a phone call and stay at the house until someone came to pick her up.

I witnessed individual fights and fights involving entire families. I experienced a young man climbing in and out of our bedroom window in the wee hours of the morning. I won't share the details of that experience because they are not mine to share. However, I will share that I was very frightened, because my bed was next to the window and the young man crawled over me.

We lived in that house for two years. We moved to Third and Shipman the summer before I started the Third grade. Although we argued a lot, there were times we actually had fun together. As we got older, we did not fight and quarrel any more, but the threats and bullying continued, and there was always an underlying tension.

At random times fights were instigated between another family member and me. This went on for a few years. Finally, the family member and I decided there was no reason for us to fight, so we decided to stop.

Growing up in a large family was a struggle. Although there were seven of us before my father married again, there seemed to be less chaos, more freedom, and more love shown. That seemed to all but dissipate after my father married again. I longed for love and attention, but I never got what I needed.

I recall as a preteen telling one of our friends I wish I had some kind of disease. She told me I just wanted some attention. She was right. Growing up in a large family, you can get lost in the mix. I got attention, but it was not the kind of attention I wanted.

Moving meant new schools and new neighbors. The school I attended was Lincoln Grade School. From Third grade to Fifth grade, I made a lot of new friends. In the Sixth grade, I met and forged a friendship with two young ladies. We became inseparable until we graduated and went to high school.

I became an aunt at the age of 9-years-old and again at the age of 12-years-old. Three years later the city bought our home, and we moved to Humboldt and Griswold. There were only a few weeks left before the school year ended, so we were allowed to finish the school year. We transferred schools at the beginning of the next school year.

One of the people I met at Lincoln Grade School was my oldest son's father. Although I had known him for years, we did not start dating until I was a sophomore in high school. I was 15-years-old at the time. Later that year, I turned 16-years-old. He had to meet my parents before we could officially date. The rule of the house for the girls was no dating until we were 16-years-old. I did not follow that rule. I snuck and dated anyway.

Because the meeting of my parents never happened, I decided to break up with my son's father. I told him if he was not "man enough" to meet my parents, he was not "man enough" to date me. My choice of words back then made me chuckle. How much of a man could he be? He was only 16-years-old.

During my junior year of high school after breaking up with my oldest son's father, I met one of my brother's friends, who was interested in dating me, so we started dating. Well, if that's what you want to call it. We went to the same school. Oh, I forgot to mention, my oldest son's father and I attended different high schools, which made it that much harder to sneak date.

My brother's friend and I wrote letters back and forth. We exchanged numbers, even though I knew I could not receive phone calls from boys. That was another rule for the girls. Sometimes when I went to choir rehearsal, I would sneak and call him before rehearsal started. On one occasion, when I made one of those calls, his mother answered the phone. She told me he wasn't there and then asked if I was the girl who kept calling her house playing on the phone. I told her no. She apologized. I was totally caught off guard by her question and felt very awkward. The next day, when I saw him at school, he apologized for the conversation between his mother and me and assured me all was well with us. I was very naïve so I believed him.

One day he called our house. I was sitting in the family room watching television. My step-mother, who was also in the family room, answered the phone. When he asked to speak to me, she told him I could not receive phone calls from boys. I got the speech about not being able to date again, which went in one ear and out the other. I did not end the relationship with my brother's friend, but after my step-mother told him I could not get phone calls from boys, he broke up with me. He would still flirt with me and be a tease, but we never got back together.

A few months later, my oldest son's father, and I got back together. He finally met my father the summer before my senior year. My step-mother was out of town at the time. At last, we were finally official.

We would go on dates every other week or when we were allowed. He had a job so we dated around paydays. We went to Homecoming my junior year, which was pretty cool. He asked me if I wanted to go to Prom my senior year. I politely declined. I am more of a tomboy so dressing in long gowns or frilly dresses don't work for me. I will wear them when I need to, but I prefer jeans and a t-shirt. My oldest son's father attended my graduation then we went out and celebrated, but I had to be home by midnight.

I found out later; he took someone else to Homecoming his junior year. I also did not get to attend his graduation. One of my sibling's graduation was the same day and time at a different school. Although I wanted to go to his graduation, I was gently persuaded to attend my sibling's graduation. Although my oldest son's father and I were the same age, we did not graduate the same year.

We had our fair share of mishaps in our relationship, which is common, but we overcame them. We dated for four years but grew apart and eventually ended our relationship.

I was 18 years old when I found out I was pregnant. I was not afraid, but I knew my life would drastically change. I knew I would have to tell my parents, but I wanted to wait. The plan was for the father and me to talk to both of our parents together. We never got the chance to tell them. As I was having a conversation with the father about who knew of my pregnancy, my younger sister just happened to walk by; she informed my step-mother before we could.

For years I thought my step-mother had extraordinary prescience, the fact of knowing something before it takes place; foreknowledge. I later learned my step-mother had the gift of discernment. My step-mother knew when I started my period. Well, that one was easy to figure out. My step-mother and I had several conversations regarding menstruation, but I was too afraid to tell her when it actually happened. So what I did was wrap up a bunch of toilet tissue and use it as a sanitary napkin. Of course, that did not work. I bled through my pants, that's how she found out.

She knew when I was pregnant. She knew when I had company when I was not supposed to and knew about me smoking marijuana. I always wondered how in the world she knew all of these things? Well, I figured it out years later. She did not know until she was told. The person that told will remain nameless.

I tried to stay out of trouble, but I received my fair share of punishments. Everyone in the family got in trouble at one time or another. Sometimes we received individual whippings other times we lined up one by one like an assembly line to receive punishment. There were several times when one individual got in trouble; they would tell on somebody else and get them in trouble. That's something I never did. What I knew I kept to myself.

Because my parents now knew I was pregnant, I knew I had to I start making plans for my baby and me. I would find a job, find an apartment, and move out. I thought if my older sister could do it, I could do it also. The only problem with that is I did not know my sister's struggle. Things aren't always as they seem. In my sister's situation, all I saw was a baby, job, apartment, not struggle. Finding a job was impossible. I applied for jobs, but I assumed because I was pregnant, no one wanted to hire me.

I graduated high school in the spring of 1982, several months before I got pregnant. A recruiter came to the house and tried to get me to sign up for the Army, which I was all for, but I was not allowed to join. Because I was 17-years-old when I graduated, I needed my parent's consent. The recruiter was vehemently told I was not joining the Army. I was going to college. I went to a junior college that fall but really did not know what I wanted to pursue. I only attended one semester, flunked out and never returned. I turned 18-years-old on my birthday later that year. The following February, I found out I was pregnant.

> Don't forget; you are human. It's okay to have a meltdown. Just don't unpack and live there. Cry it out. Then refocus on where you are headed.
> **Bill Barr**

Throughout my pregnancy, I felt I totally disappointed and shamed my family. I always seemed to do something that caused my parents to lecture me. I felt bad enough as it was, but it seemed like every week there was something.

While carrying my baby, all I could think about was I just want someone to love and someone to love me unconditionally. I didn't plan to get pregnant, but I also didn't do anything to prevent it.

One Sunday before our afternoon service started, I went to the basement of the church where several youth choir members were and announced I was pregnant. I did it in jest not thinking anybody was paying attention to me. They were. One of the choir members inquired about my announcement.

It got back to my parents, who in turn gave me a very long lecture. I knew me having sex out of wedlock was wrong, and the pregnancy was the consequence, but me making that announcement was a cry for attention. I wasn't the first one to have a baby out of wedlock, but it seemed like my pregnancy disgraced the family.

I had never been pregnant before, but because I felt I messed up and could not ask for help, I tried to do everything on my own. That was not true; it was how I felt at the time. My misguided perception of things.

I was almost seven months pregnant before I got prenatal care. Not because I didn't want to, it took that long to get an appointment at the clinic. I didn't want to be a burden to my parents, so I applied for a few jobs. As I said earlier, nobody wanted to hire a pregnant woman. Since I could not find work, I hung out and did nothing. I went on a few dates with the father, but that's about it besides attending church. With some prodding from my step-mother, I signed up to get Public Aid. I also applied for subsidized housing.

It was a long summer. My hormones were all over the place. I got into several arguments with my oldest son's father and my family over small things. One of the disputes with the father was about being a few minutes late to see a movie. Yeah, I know, silly. We planned to go to see a show earlier that week. I researched and found out where and what time the movie was to start. The day came for us to go. The movie started at 7:00 p.m. I sat patiently waiting for the father to pick me up. He finally arrived about ten minutes before the show was to start. I was mad. When I got into his truck, I did not say a word. He broke the speed limit to get us to the theatre. Because it was after 7:00 p.m., I refused to get out of his truck. He went in to see if the movie started. When he came back to tell me the movie was about two minutes in, I ignored him and still would not get out of the truck. He conceded and took me back home.

The ride home was quiet. He tried to talk to me, but I would not speak to him. When we got to my house, I exited the truck quickly and went into the house without saying goodbye, see you later or anything. He got out of the truck and followed me into the house, pleading with me to talk to him. I refused to speak to him, which made him angry. He left my house in a huff and went home. We did not talk for days.

After a week or so, we finally started talking again. I do not remember who called who but we were back in effect. A couple of months later, I began hearing rumors about him seeing someone else. It was gossip, so I did not put too much stock in what was being said. Of course, he denied it. I soon found out the rumors were true, and I was being cheated on. While dating this other girl, he impregnated her. She ended up losing the baby, but that's beside the point. Because he kept denying he was cheating, my sister and I played a trick on him. She called him pretending to be the other girl. She mentioned something about being pregnant. He responded by saying he thought she lost the baby. She told him she did not lose the baby after all. That's all I needed to hear. Rumor confirmed. Turns out he was dating a girl that was the sister of my cousin's girlfriend. Small world and the city we live in is even smaller. Chances are someone will know you or know of you, yet you have never met. I was hurt but hid my pain. Trust was broken. I thought we had something special.

Although I busted him cheating on me while I was pregnant, I didn't break up with him. I chose to stay. I am positive he never stopped cheating, but I could not prove it. I resolved to have the baby and deal with the cheating after the baby was born.

My baby was born in the fall of that year. I had to grow up pretty fast because I now had a little one to take care of. I was still living in my parent's home. I had not been called for an apartment yet. I am grateful for the time I was there because I knew nothing about how to take care of a baby. Seven months later I received a call for an apartment in the Warner Homes. I was ecstatic. Finally, I could move out on my own and get from under all of those rules. After I moved out, I said I would never come back home. I had to eat those words a year or so later.

A few months after moving out of my parent's house, I stopped dating my oldest son's biological father. We grew apart. I didn't trust him. However, before our relationship ended, I got him back for cheating on me. Yep. That was my plan all along. After I cheated, I called him and told him. I acted as if I regretted it. I cried and everything. It was all an act. I wanted him to feel what I felt when I found out he cheated on me. He was angry, but I didn't care.

A few months later, I started dating the man I would eventually marry. We actually met while we were still in high school. We went to different schools, but the summer before my senior year we both got jobs with the Youth Conservation Cooperation. Our first day on the job everyone reported to Forrest Park Nature Center. That is where I first saw him. We were assigned to different crews, so that was the only day we worked together. We did not see each other again until after we both graduated from high school. By then, I was living on my own with a child.

A friend of his attended the same church I did so from time to time they would ride their bikes to the church and hang out. One day I was getting ready to walk to choir rehearsal, we lived within walking distance of the church. He and his friend rode their bikes to our house. His friend liked my sister. She walked with me. My sister and his friend were chatting while my future husband and I awkwardly waited until they finished their conversation. They rode their bikes to the church often. Sometimes on a choir rehearsal day, others times after service on Sunday.

One Sunday after service, his friend asked me out of the blue if I liked my future husband. I didn't recall who he was speaking of at first until he described him. I told him I would have to meet him and then decide. We officially met one night after going the Heart of Illinois Fair. We were with my future husband's friend, who I later found out was my cousin. After we left the fair, we went riding around and saw my future husband parked in a lot, so we stopped. We talked for a minute; then I went home.

My future husband and I started dating after that meeting. He was right for me. Before I met him, even though I wanted more, I was content getting a check, food stamps, and living in the projects. He showed me I could do better and be better. He encouraged me to think differently and challenged me to find a job. I applied for and got a summer job through the Urban League. I didn't have a car at the time, so I took the bus. Every morning I would get on the bus with my son, ride to the south end of town to drop him off at my parent's house, then get back on the bus and ride it downtown to the courthouse where I worked for the summer. After that job ended, I applied for another position. Once I found a job, I got off Public Aid and bought a car. That gave me a little more freedom to move around.

I worked for a few months then decided I wanted to get out of Peoria. I saved money to purchase a plane ticket for my son and me, who was 2-years-old at the time. I booked our flights, gave notice at my job and flew out to Los Angeles, California to start a new life.

One of my older brothers and his family lived in Pomona, California. He and his wife allowed us to live with them. When I got there, it didn't take me long to find a job. I knew my son, and I would not be able to live with my brother and his family forever, so I started planning again. I planned to buy a car then find an apartment, so I started saving money. I sent a letter to the Peoria Housing Authority informing them to cancel my lease. However, after living in California for a month, I realized I did not like it as much as I thought I would, so I decided to move back to Peoria. I gave two weeks' notice at my place of employment and planned to leave at the end of the two weeks. Due to circumstances beyond my control that I won't go in to, my son and I had to leave earlier than planned. I bought bus tickets for both of us, and we left immediately. It was a long ride back to my hometown, three days to be exact. Though it was a tough decision to come back home, I'm glad I did. California was not for me.

After returning to Peoria, I moved back in with my parents. My step-mother told me I still had my apartment. I am forever grateful that she called the Peoria Housing Authority on my behalf and asked them not to cancel my lease.

A month or so later, I was encouraged to move back to my apartment. Once I left that time, I never went back. I re-established myself, found a job, bought another car, and continued raising my son on my own. I found a third shift job, which meant I needed to be able to sleep during the day.

With a two-year-old, that was not easy. I worked that job for a few months; then I applied again to the company where I was employed before I moved to California. They rehired me in a different position. A few months later I left my apartment in the Warner Homes and moved to Hedgehill Apartments. I bought another car, applied for and was accepted at Midstate College. I continued working while attending college.

I made the Dean's List every quarter and graduated with honors as a Court Reporter's Assistant. After graduating, I continued working at my current place of employment. About a year or so later, I was sitting in my bedroom one afternoon, thinking about my future. I liked the job I had, but I wanted to start a career. The Holy Spirit reminded me that the college I attended had a lifetime employment placement program. I called the school and spoke with someone who gave me a referral for the Social Security Administration. God opened the door for me to be hired in a temporary position that lasted four years. I was laid off for six weeks then rehired in a permanent position. The Lord answered my prayer without me uttering one word. *Now to Him who is able to do exceedingly abundantly above all that we ask or think, according to the power that works in us (Ephesians 3:20 NKJV)*

My hubby and I dated for six years before we got married. I was determined not to have any more children until then. I still was not doing things the right way, and I believe the only reason I didn't get pregnant is that I was taking birth control. I knew I should not be having sex before marriage, but I wanted to please my flesh more than please God. I was still attending service, singing in the choir and fornicating. The examples I had before me made me think it was okay because they were believers as well. We should be careful about the life we live because you never know who is watching.

It wasn't until we decided to get married that I began to listen to the Holy Spirit who convicted me about having sex before marriage. I read the book Marriage and the Family by Frederick K. Price. Although it was for married couples, I read it for insight. There was a small section in the book for singles. While reading that section, the one thing that stuck out to me the most was abstaining from sex until marriage. I was immediately convicted. I also heard a sermon shortly after reading the book that addressed the same thing. I surrendered to God and stopped having sex. That became a challenge in my relationship. My husband, who was my boyfriend at the time, didn't understand why we had to stop. We had been sexually active for years. Why stop now. We decided to get married that same year, so I told him I wanted to do it right and wait. We stopped for a while, but I eventually gave in a few weeks before we were married. Instead of me trying to rely on my strength, I should have asked God to give me the strength to abstain.

After we were married for a year or so, I stopped taking the pill because I no longer wanted to put anything foreign in my body. I discussed it with my husband first. About six months later, we were pregnant. My second son was born the following year.

My babies are a blessing from God. They are unique in their particular way. My oldest is outgoing, popular, smart, funny, giving, compassionate, and has many other outstanding traits. My youngest is more laid back, popular, intelligent, funny, caring, and kind and also has many other exceptional characteristics. They are both loving husbands and great fathers, and I am honored to have been chosen to be their mother.

CHAPTER 2

Uncovering the Shadow
"The Lie, This Is Who I Am."

Ipersonally never used that lie. The lie I used was just that, a lie. "I'm a realist." That's what I tell people. You won't get fake here. I don't do fake people. Truth is, I was a fake. To borrow lyrics from a song from Dreamgirls titled "Fake Your Way to the Top", I was faking my way through life. I didn't even like who I was. When I looked in the mirror, all I saw was hurt, rejection, molestation, rape, guilt, and shame, and that's what defined me.

I was a broken little girl living in a grown woman's body. On some days, I was the three-year-old, longing for her mother or the broken seven-year-old wanting attention. On other days I was the 12-year-old trying to fit in or the 15-year-old who just wanted to be left alone. Still other days the 17-year old wishing the molestation and rape would finally end.

"Sometimes, God will break your spirit to save your soul." Pastor Kimberly Jones-Pothier

When I was 12 years old, I struggled to find myself. It was an awkward time for me. At that age you're not a little kid anymore but, you're also not a teenager. You struggle to fit in and find your identity. I didn't quite fit in at school or home. As I stated at the beginning of this book, my mother and father had seven children, six boys, and one girl. I was the youngest of the bunch. My mother passed away when I was three years old, leaving my dad to raise seven children on his own. Being a man, he could handle the boys, but he did not know how to teach a girl to be a woman. After speaking with a friend of the family in 2018, she told my father decided to marry a woman who had girls so she could teach me how to be a woman. Along with learning how to be a woman, I was introduced to sex through my molesters.

I was molested from the age of 12 years old until I was 17 years old. I do not understand why it happened, and I never questioned it. I just wanted it to stop. Although I wanted to, I never exposed the perpetrators. I told myself if I allowed it, maybe the perpetrators would like me. I know, sounds weird. But I now understand I needed affection, attention and just wanted to be loved.

"All girls need healthy and consistent love to become healthy and consistent women" Iyanla Vanzant.

In the basement of the house on Third and Shipman, there were several rooms. The front area is where the washing machine was located. We did not own a Whirlpool or Maytag; we had an old fashioned wringer washer. We did not own a dryer at that time either. We hung our clothes on the clothesline in our back yard.

By the age of 12-years-old, I was responsible for washing my clothes. One wash day I was in the basement washing my clothes. I was running my clothes through the wringer, which you had to do one piece at a time when the perpetrator came down the stairs. The perpetrator walked past me; I thought he was coming downstairs to feed the dogs, so I did not give his presence a second thought. I continued wringing my clothes out. I felt hands on my butt; then his body pressed up against me. I didn't know what was happening and was too afraid to look. He told me to go into one of the back rooms. I learned as a child to keep the peace I had to conform, so I complied. There was a ledge attached to the wall large enough for me to lay on. He told me to lie down, then he got on top of me and pleasured his self. We didn't remove our clothing, that would come much later. When he was done, he went back upstairs. I got up, went back into the room where the washer was and continued wringing my clothes out. After I finished wringing my clothes out, I took them outside and hung them on the clothesline. I acted as if nothing happened. I never told anyone. I was too afraid.

After that first encounter in the basement, if I was ever alone in the house and the perpetrator was there, more often than not, I would get molested again. No place in the house was safe from the perpetrator. About a year or so later, the second perpetrator started sexually violating me.

On rare occasions, we were allowed to stay at home while my parents went to church. One particular evening, the house was quiet. Everyone was either in their room or gone. I was laying on the couch in the family room next to the window, relaxing. I had my eyes closed. I thought I heard someone creeping down the stairs, but I did not open my eyes. I felt someone get on top of me and start grinding. My body tensed. I did not move; I did not open my eyes; I did not try to fight him off. When he finished, he went back upstairs. Relief, or so I thought. A few minutes later, the second perpetrator crept down the stairs and got on top of me and start grinding. I let my body go limp until he finished and went back upstairs. I laid there for a minute, then decided that spot wasn't safe anymore, in case they wanted to creep back down the stairs again. I got up quickly and went upstairs to the bedroom I shared with the other girls. I felt like I was just a piece of meat to be used for someone else's pleasure. Because of how my body was used, I started hating it. I hated everything about my body. My forehead was too big; my eyes were too big, my legs were too skinny. My feet were ugly, my breasts were small, and I did not have a butt. Even after my body developed, I still hated it. That hate would carry into adulthood and affect the way I viewed myself inside and out.

Something else I hated was my middle name. I loved my first name, Juanita and cherished my maiden name Thornton, but I detested my middle name. I thought it was the ugliest name ever. My middle name is Rezella. In my mind, it was similar to Cruella and Medusa. I found out in my early 30s that Rezella is my biological mother's middle name. I still thought it was ugly.

Besides having her middle name, I always wondered what my life would be like or how different it would be if my biological mother were still alive. Would I have experienced molestation, rejection, or bullying? Would I have experienced some other kind of dysfunction? Would I have a happy life or one full of strife?

Because I knew so little about her as a person, I often wondered if I was anything like her. Do I have any of her traits? Do I act like her in any kind of way? What was she like? A lot of facts were shared with me regarding my mother like her mother died giving birth to her. My mother was raised by a step-mother and step-father. She had three brothers and a sister. I was told by several people who knew my mother that she was sweet and kind. This information was great, but it was not enough. I knew I looked like her, but even that was not enough. I needed at least one thing I could cherish since I did not have her.

I was proud to have her middle name, but I did not like it. When people would ask me what the "R" stood for and I would tell them, they would say, that is beautiful. I would smile and say thanks, but in my head, I was saying, "Yeah, right."

My mother loved her middle name. She even signed her yearbook with it. I longed to have something I could cherish from my mother. It took me over 40 years to embrace my middle name. I finally realized, after 52 years, she gave me something that she cherished, her middle name. It is an honor to have my mother's middle name, and I will cherish it forever.

Another thing I cherished was the brief time the molestation stopped. One of the perpetrators and I were punished for what my parents thought was inappropriate behavior between us. That is why the molestation stopped. What they did not know is I never wanted the molestation to happen. It was forced upon me. Unfortunately, about six months or so later it started again. Because I had no control over the molestation and abuse, I felt powerless. Trust was broken. How come the adults in the house did not recognize what was going on? Why didn't they dig deeper and see past the shell of a person I was becoming? Couldn't they look in my eyes, the window to my soul, and realize I was hurting?

Because I felt I had no control while growing up, I try to control everything in my life as much as I can now. I do not allow people to get close to me because of trust issues. If I let you get close to me, that means I trust you but not completely. I still will not let you get close enough to hurt me. I keep everybody at arm's length. Trying to be in control of everything wears you out and causes you to be trapped and not be able to move forward.

I was listening to a sermon by Pastor Michael Todd of Transformation Church, and in his message, he said, "The formula to forgetting your past is fixed focus. Our focus should be on Jesus." He then asked, "Where are you fixing your focus?" The molestation caused me to carry a lot of things that weighed me down. I internalized everything. The bullying, being shunned, molestation, rejection, marginalization, and church hurt. For years my focus was fixed on the guilt and shame that came from the molestation and abuse. I lived every day in fear. I never wanted to be alone in a room with a male for fear that they may try to molest or abuse me. Whenever I had any kind of encounter with a male, and they did anything that I thought was inappropriate, I automatically assumed they wanted to have sex with me. I forgave the perpetrators years ago, but for me to move forward, I have to fully let go of the past, fix my focus on Jesus and what's ahead.

As you will read in the following chapters, The Fallacy of Perfection, Disregard, Rejection, Spirit of Comparison, Insignificance, Search for Significance, and Girl Behind the Veil were lies the devil sold me. I bought the lies, put them in a suitcase, and unpacked them when I felt the need to. They were my comfort zone. As long as I stayed in that zone, I could use the lies as an excuse if I acted out of character, the mental and moral qualities distinctive to an individual.

For me to act out of character, I have to know my character traits. If you were to ask me to describe myself, I would probably tell you I am patient, stubborn, compassionate, sarcastic, dependable; I love to laugh and love to make people laugh. That's not how others describe me as you will read in a later chapter.

Continuing to uncover the shadow of the lie this is who I am, it's funny how people think they actually know you. Recalling a conversation with an associate some years back, she commented that she knew me. I listened to her but chuckled inside. I thought to myself, you think you know me, but you don't. To begin with, we weren't that close. We hung out a few times. She was cool, but I never let my guard down when we were together. In an attempt to open up a little, I decided to share something personal about my childhood. From that one conversation, she concluded that she knew me. Boy was she wrong. What she knew was the mask I wore.

I don't like being around a lot of people. If I could control the number of people I came in contact with, then I could control how well they got to know me. I could give them the surface me and never go more in-depth. Unfortunately, that did not work all of the time. In reality, I didn't know me. I wore several masks, and because I didn't know myself, I would say this is how God made me. I mean He must have, He allowed all this mess to happen to me. I later said He allowed me to be broken so I can help others. I learned later that, that part is true, but I didn't understand that at the time. Everything He allows is working for my good and His glory. It took me 52 years to realize that truth. After learning that truth, I asked God to show me who He created me to be. I also asked Him to show me my purpose, so I can walk in it and fulfill the plan He has for my life. Having compassion is part of that plan. My father was very humble and compassionate. God has given me compassion for people as well.

My heart bleeds for people, but I will not allow their hearts to ache for me. For that to happen, I have to trust them enough to let them get close to me. I genuinely love people and want the best for them, but I try to keep them at arm's length. If I allowed them in, they would see how jacked up I was and the façade of a life I was living. Our connection had to stay at the surface level. We sometimes went into shallow waters, but we hardly ever went under water, and we never went deep. I wouldn't allow it. With my spiritual daughters, it's totally different. We actually do life together. There are still some areas we are not privy to in each other's lives, and that's ok. I love my spiritual daughters, just like they are my own.

CHAPTER 3

Unteachable, Not Me, I'm Always Willing to Learn

God uses the most unlikely objects to teach you a lesson. I was awake in the wee hours of the morning Super Bowl Sunday 2019. No matter how hard I tried, I could not go back to sleep. In 2017, I attended a grief share potluck. As I stated earlier, my biological mother passed away in 1967 when I was three years old. I was still grieving because I never got to know her. I was also still grieving my father, who was my everything.

Ok so back to the most unlikely objects. The need to use the restroom awakened me. Before I got out of bed, a person came to mind that occasionally rubbed me the wrong way. My way of coping with that is to ignore them. I was good at ignoring people or acting as if they did not exist. Something I learned as a child.

I cried out to God and asked why I treated this person as if they didn't exist at times. After using the restroom, I washed my hands and reached for the towel to dry my hands. When I grabbed it, the hanger fell. This was not the first time it had fallen, but this time, I said to myself, "This thing needs to be replaced." I looked at the towel hanger and asked God, "What does this have to do with that person?" I pleaded with God and asked if there is something I need to learn from this person? Is there something in me that I recognize in them? Nope, it was not about them at all. It was about me. I am one of several directors at my place of worship. I teach songs as well. I asked God years ago, when He gave me the desire to direct, to enhance my ear so I can teach songs as well. This person had an ear to hear music and would sometimes question what I was teaching. Other people did this also, but the difference was, I took it as an offense from this person. I even viewed it as a competition. In my mind, I thought they could not teach me anything. God showed me through a towel hanger that I saw myself as irreplaceable.

Google Dictionary's definition of irreplaceable is: impossible to replace if lost or damaged. Synonyms: unique, unrepeatable, incomparable, unparalleled, priceless, invaluable, beyond price, without price, inestimably precious, of incalculable value/worth, or inestimable value/worth, or immeasurable value/worth, worth its weight in gold, treasured, prized, cherished.

I chuckled when I saw the synonyms of irreplaceable. Yes, I am unique; we all are. But I'm not so amazing that I can't be replaced. God showed me I viewed myself that way a few times. Mostly I was saying without verbally saying it, "God You can't use nobody else the way You use me." Really Juanita! Full of pride is what I was. It was rooted so deep in me, God had to excavate and extract it. *Pride goes before destruction and haughtiness before a fall. (Proverbs 16:18 NLT)* God showed me, by using that towel hanger, that I did see myself that way, and it was rooted in pride because of rejection and the need for acceptance.

I had to humble myself to be teachable. God had to show me that someone else could also hear, teach, and direct, and it had nothing to do with competing with me. I asked for forgiveness, then asked God to do whatever He needed to do to make me the woman He created me to be and that included performing surgery on me. Just as with most operations, with the extraction came pain.

CHAPTER 4

Tearing Down the Fallacy of Perfection

I always want to get things right. There nothing wrong with that until I make a mistake.

As a child, when I became a conformer, I tried to do everything right. I strived to please my step-mother. I tried to follow the rules, do as I was told, and stay out of trouble. I followed the rules because I didn't like getting into trouble. I wanted to show her how much she was appreciated. I knew I couldn't get everything right all of the time, but I tried. Whether at home, at school, at church, or wherever, if given a task, I wanted to do it right. I didn't know me trying to do everything right would lead to becoming a perfectionist.

Trying to be perfect started out innocent. Not realizing it, I carried striving for perfection into adulthood, and it became a challenge for me.

I started taking piano lessons as an adult. My mother and step-mother played the piano, and I wanted to learn how to play as well. At one of my sessions, I was plucking away at the notes and tried to play them correctly, but I kept messing up so instead of continuing to play, I would go back and re-play it. The teacher said to me, "You're a perfectionist. It's ok to make a mistake, you're learning." I was a little embarrassed because I wanted to play the song right, but I didn't. I never thought of myself as being a perfectionist, but the more I self-evaluated I could see how she saw that in me.

Google Dictionary's definition of perfection is the action or process of improving something until it is faultless or as fault-less as possible.

Now on the surface, that sounds great. Nothing wrong with wanting things to be right. It becomes dangerous when you're trying to be perfect for the wrong reasons.

After learning my piano teacher thought I was a perfec-tionist, I had to do some soul-searching. I never saw myself as being a perfectionist, and I certainly never thought anyone else had those thoughts about me. I soon learned differently.

I am a singer. I believe if you're going to minister in song, properly studying your craft is essential, but removing yourself and allowing the anointing of the Holy Spirit is vital. I love singing; it's my passion. I also enjoy studying music and learning the songs, so I made sure I studied regularly. When I started directing choirs, I asked God to enhance my ear to hear the different parts (soprano, alto, tenor) in songs. At my current place of worship, we have several praise teams and a choir. I have the privilege of singing on the praise team and in the choir. Because I love to study music, after I learn the so-prano part, I could usually pick up alto and tenor as well. At times while going over songs in rehearsal if someone didn't have their part, they would ask me. Sometimes I could give the part, sometimes I couldn't, so I would listen to the song again and try to sing it. Then there were times the notes were not executed right, and I knew it so I would give it without being asked. This was well-received sometimes, other times it seemed to be problematic. When we ministered on Sundays, if the parts weren't right, it would show on my face.

I was chastised about my facial expressions several times, so to rectify that, I started acting as if I didn't know the other parts. I was chastised for this, too, so singing began to become a sore spot for me. I still love to sing, and I always strive for excellence, but my focus is not so much on notes/parts but an audience of one, our Heavenly Father.

Over the years, we've had many music ministry meetings. One of our meetings was at a restaurant. I don't remember what it was about, but everyone was allowed to share their thoughts and concerns. When it was my turn, I started by saying, "I was told I was a perfectionist." Before I could say anything else, I was rebuked and told I was not perfect and everybody makes mistakes. The person who rebuked said a whole lot more. I really can't remember everything, but I was totally caught off guard. I had no idea they felt that way about me. I never thought I was perfect and never thought me striving to get things right came across that way.

Taking self-inventory, I have to confess if I make a mistake, which is inevitable, I try to justify it. I notice that about me more so in the workplace. Instead of owning up to the fact that I overlooked or just did not do what I was supposed to do, I look for a reason to explain why I did not do my part. Either I did not get the right information, or I cannot do what I am supposed to do if the person I am doing it for has not done their part. All of this stems from wanting to be the perfect little girl for my step-mother to show her how much she was appreciated.

Perfectionism is rooted in pride. It was a pride-fueled effort to win approval. Yes, I wanted to show appreciation, but I also did not want to be rejected, so I tried to be perfect. *For do I now persuade men or God? Or do I seek to please men? For if I still pleased men, I would not be a bondservant of Christ. (Galatians 1:10 NKJV)*

Perfectionism is something I could never achieve because we all fall short. Unfortunately, my pride fueled attempt to win approval for me carried on into adulthood. Still seeking the acceptance of others who could care less about me. *Therefore, since we are surrounded by such a huge crowd of witnesses to the life of faith, let us strip off every weight that slows us down, especially the sin that so easily trips us up. And let us run with endurance the race God has set before us (Hebrews 12:1 NLT)* I am still discovering those things that are buried deep inside me in my effort to become whole. This journey is not effortless, but I am pressing my way through.

CHAPTER 5

The Damage of Rejection

While reading about Uprooting Insecurity in Pastor Toure' Roberts book Wholeness, he challenges the reader to find the feeling that insecurity causes. His definition of insecurity is evidence of a negative, untrue, and devaluing thought. Mine was the feeling of being disregarded.

When I was between the ages of nine and eleven years old, I had a chance to march in the Santa Claus Parade, a tradition that takes place downtown in our city every year the day after Thanksgiving. Several children were going to perform a routine during the parade. I was excited. I attended all of the practices in preparation for that particular day. I made sure I paid attention to and remembered the time we were to meet at Carver Community Center before we went to the parade. When the day arrived, I was at the Community Center early. One of the leaders started choosing the children who would be marching. Your attendance at practice determined who would be selected. I watched in anticipation as each child was called forward. I didn't get chosen because the leader said I was not at the practices. I tried to tell the leader I did fulfill the requirement. One of the other leaders also spoke up on my behalf, but he ignored both of us. That leader chose people who had not attended all of the practices as required. I was devastated, so I went home and told my stepmother what happened. She told me to go back to the Community Center and inform the leader I was at the practices. I told her I had already done that. She did not respond but kept doing what she was doing. Those interactions caused me to think no one valued me or my what I said. It also made me not trust those in authority.

I grew up in a blended family with lots of personalities to deal with. I was one of the youngest, so we were just kind of there. Although there were girls in the house, it did not make things any easier for me. I dealt with rejection, bullying, being shunned, molestation, and rape. I would get taken advantage of regularly. I would get threatened and talked about on a regular too. I was made to do things I did not want to do. For the sake of peace. I went along with it.

With so many people in the house, you could easily get overlooked. I kept to myself a lot. I would stay in my room or sit and watch television while everyone else was out doing their thing. I didn't want to make waves, so I pretty much tried to stay out of the way. There were times that I loved being outside, running, playing volleyball with the neighbors or whatever other game we came up, those were fun times. But they only lasted for a little while; then it was back to the reality of being alone. Imagine being in a room full of people, but yet you still feel alone. That's how I felt the majority of my life. Sometimes I still experience feelings of loneliness.

I did my chores as expected and tried to do them well. I was a rule follower. I always said rules are made to be followed, so I attempted to comply with all of them. I did not like getting punished.

I remember one day we got our report cards. I did not particularly like the grades that I received, I thought I had done a better job than what I actually did, but I had to give my report card to my parents anyway. When I got home, I went up to my room, put my stuff down, and handed my report card to my step-mother. She took it, looked at it, then turned and walked away from me and made a comment that made me feel worse than I already did. I was already embarrassed about the grades. In my mind, I failed her again. Recall, I was trying to be perfect for her.

There was another time as a teenager we were watching the premiere of the Michael Jackson video Thriller. Back then, they didn't play videos all day as they do now. The videos were shown at certain times. A family member came in just as the video was going off. They wanted to know when the video would play again. I watched closely to see when the next showing would be and told them. Well, the next day, I got fussed out because the video did not come on at the time that I said it would. I was told I think I know everything and called a "Miss Know It All" when all I was trying to do was help out. The video did actually play at the time I said it would, just not Central time. The time I told the family member was Eastern time. At that time, I did not fully understand Eastern, Central, Mountain, or Pacific time. I thought it was the same time everywhere.

I wanted so bad to fit in and be liked by the people I grew up with. I felt as though I could never quite do things right. I tried not to be disrespectful and pretty much obeyed the rules most of the time. If I did not, there would be consequences to pay. I did not mind following rules, but when others didn't follow them, and there were no consequences for their disobedience, it angered me. Because I didn't like getting punished, I tried to master the art of compliance.

Google Dictionary's definition of compliance is the action or fact of complying with a wish or command.

Trying to be compliant can cause relationship issues. If you have problems with your father, it can cause relationship issues with God. My problem was, did I really trust that God would take care of me. My father was physically present (meaning he lived in the household), but he was never physically present when he was home. There was no family time, no daddy-daughter time; we saw each other in passing like two ships passing in the night. On the rare occasion we spoke, it was most likely when I brought him his dinner. I was responsible for making sure his plate was fixed and set aside for when he finally came home. The other occasion was when he chastised me. I remember as a teenager exchanging words with my Dad (sassing as the elders would say) and him calling me fast, another term the elders used when a young lady smarted off at the mouth, which is what I was brave enough to do at the time. The elders also called you fast if you gave a young man too much attention. I did not like being called that word, so I never got smart with him again.

Being compliant can affect your relationship with your siblings and how you see Jesus. He is the son of God; we are God's children, that makes Jesus our brother. You love your siblings, but sometimes you don't want to deal with them. You love Jesus, but sometimes you feel even though he was tempted and had struggles, he could never understand yours.

Then Jesus was led by the Spirit into the wilderness to be tempted there by the devil (Matthew 4:1 NLT)

Having issues with your mother because of compliance can cause you to see the Holy Spirit different. I know in my head the Holy Spirit is here with me, but I sometimes struggle in my heart to believe she is present. Because my biological mother abandoned me through death, and my father abandoned me emotionally, I struggled with the belief that the Holy Spirit is with me all the time, especially when I can not hear her clearly.

When you have the mindset of compliance, you are celebrated, you get attention and recognition, and you won't get punished because you follow the rules. You may not like the rules, but you obey them because you are told to. You are one of those people who don't cause trouble. You are like a robot with no heart, no spirit, no soul. God doesn't want robots he wants children that bare His image.

Being compliant and being a perfectionist went hand in hand for me. If I tried to be the perfect child and did as I was told, maybe I would be accepted.

At one of our rehearsals, I got into an argument over hair texture. I felt horrible afterward. I also thought about that silly argument way too long, which means it bothered me. After some reflection on why pondering on that ridiculous argument so long bothered me, I realized:

I didn't have to challenge the comment that was made about good hair.

Because I did, I could have commented in the form of a question instead of making a statement.

When I felt challenged, I did not have to rise to the challenge. I should have conceded before it turned into an argument.

I used to be happy and free before my father remarried. After reading another chapter in Wholeness and contemplating on what I read, I realized why I did not concede my sense of self and my voice. It all started when I was seven-years-old. Because my voice was shut down so often while growing up, when I feel it's being shut down now, I lash back. Sometimes out of anger, because I revert to that seven-year-old whose voice was taken from her. The result of that is, I'm not going to let anybody talk over me or keep me silent. Because of this, it sometimes leads to conflict. I hate conflict of any kind, so I don't do well in those situations. Oh yeah, I use sarcasm a lot too. Using sarcasm is another way to mask my true feelings.

I had an amazingly fulfilling moment with God the night before that silly argument happened. I was overwhelmed by His presence. That night of the debate, I asked God to give me a moment like He did the previous night.

I was diagnosed with narcolepsy in 2008, so I don't sleep well, and sleep is precious to me. I was diagnosed in 2018 with sleep apnea, which means I stop breathing while sleeping. I also snore. Because my husband was concerned about the way I was snoring, he woke me up. I tried to go back to sleep but couldn't. Earlier that night, I read Regina's story in the book Wholeness. It was almost midnight when I got a revelation of why I got into that silly argument.

I got involved in community theatre in 2014. During my very first show, a person made the comment that I had nappy hair. I don't think the intent was to cause harm. It may have been their perception of what a woman of color hair is like. Because I didn't know them personally, I did not respond, but I was offended. A few years later, I was in another show; this person made a comment again. This time I did say something, not directly to them because I was speaking with another person about how they wanted me to wear my hair for the upcoming show, but loud enough for them to hear me say my hair is curly, not nappy. Yes, that was a passive-aggressive response. What I should have done was addressed and educated the person who made a comment the first time it was made. I didn't realize how deeply that comment offended me until now.

The Holy Spirit also reminded me that I am on a journey, and in the book Wholeness, Pastor Toure' said it would get worse before it gets better. The Holy Spirit also revealed to me why I felt horrible after that meaningless argument. I have a great relationship with the person, they are like a little sister in Christ to me, and I really do love them. Otherwise, it wouldn't have bothered me much. I'm on a journey to get whole. Still, so much work to be done and that jerk Satan will continue to test and distract me. But I am victorious because of Christ. He set me free, and I am whole in Him. The journey continues.

CHAPTER 6

Spirit of Comparison

Comparison is without wisdom. Each call is unique - Stephanie Ike

I am grateful for the gift of exhortation the Lord has given me, and the talent to exhort through song. As I stated earlier, singing is my passion. I absolutely love it.

I have loved singing since I was a little girl. I would make songs up just to sing. I could sing 24 hours a day 7 days a week and never get tired, that's how much I love it.

I started out singing in the Sunshine Band at the church where my Father was the Pastor. I remember belting out the notes as loud as I could and loving it. I love hearing melodies and harmonies, the beat of the drum, the rumble of the bass and sweet sound of the organ all working together. It soothes my soul. It wasn't until I was an adult that I started noticing this comparison thing. I have been at churches, different events or around people that would make comments or encourage individual singers but tend to overlook the gift/talent of other singers because that particular singer's voice may not be as versatile.

I started to let that affect me in ways that I cannot put into words. I know what the Lord has given me, but I started telling myself that I wasn't as good as other singers and nobody wanted to hear me. I tend to devalue the gift and talents God has given me more often than not (e.g., I was asked to sing at an event. My immediate thought was if so and so was still living here I would not have been approached.) I let the accolades and comments about other singers affect me so much so, I started shying away from invitations to sing with community choirs or groups.

I am in no way saying I'm the greatest singer of all time nor do I even come close but, I do have a wonderful gift and talent that the Lord entrusted me with and I definitely want to use it to glorify Him. Unfortunately, I found myself trying to mimic other singers, which caused me to devalue the uniqueness of my God-given talent. It didn't matter how many accolades I was given; I would always downplay them.

I have to confess there were times I secretly wanted the accolades. Most of the time, when I would receive compliments, I would humbly defer the gratitude to God. When I didn't receive them, I would start speculating and conclude I must not be good enough to get them. Because I am an artist, I continually ask myself, am I looking for applause or recognition? Am I seeking validation from man? Is my identity in my works or God?

While speaking with one of my best friends one day, she shared with me that the Lord was asking her these questions. I thought about what God was asking her and had to do some self-inventory. I can honestly say, I do seek applause and recognition at times, and I also seek validation in various areas of my life. She told me the last thing God said to her was the validation you look for from a man you will never find. That statement hit me hard. It took many years for me to realize that no matter how hard I try to please and appease people, it will never be enough. The reason I sought to please and appease man is that I wanted validation from them. That would be impossible because man is not God. He is the only one who can validate me.

I have come to appreciate the gift and talent the Lord has given me. It's unique because I am unique. What God gave me is for me, and however He wants to use me in that area, I am willing and ready to be used. What we have to remember and understand is God gave each of us our very own unique gift and talent. He has called each of us in one capacity or another. Even if our call is in the same area, it is still different from mine. There is room for everybody. God uniquely made us in His Holy image. God is still working on me in that area. Sometimes I forget and fall back into the comparison trap. There is no need for comparison. You undermine your potential when you compare yourself to someone else.

Singing is not the only area I compared myself to others. I was given the nickname "Skinny Legs and All." From as far back as I can remember, I was called that nickname by one of my babysitters. I don't think she meant any harm by giving me that nickname, but it caused me to have a complex about my legs as well. When I was about 7 or 8 years old, I was outside playing in the dirt by myself. It was summertime, so I had shorts on. For some reason, I looked at my legs and thought, "Hmmm, my legs ain't skinny, they are pretty." I took pride in how my legs were shaped and how smooth they were; I even liked the color. I was really into my legs. To put it into perspective, I thought about my legs, the way others thought about Tina Turner's legs. I thought they were just that cute, and I started to become prideful about my legs. I had a great aunt who was tall, voluptuous and had big calves. She had a very commanding presence. One day she came to visit, I looked at her calves and said to myself, "I hope my calves don't look like that when I grow up." Now why I said that I have no idea because her calves weren't overly huge, they fit her body and shape. While I was prideful about my legs, I was judging hers. Not too long after that, I caught the chickenpox, and my legs were ruined with scars from the bumps. I never looked at my legs the same.

Even as a little girl, I would compare myself to other little girls. I didn't know how to see myself differently. The older I got, the more I compared myself. I was tall and skinny with long arms and long legs. I didn't start developing until I was in the 8th grade. That is the year I started wearing a real bra. I had on a shirt that kind of accentuated my breasts. I was walking home from school one spring day. When I got to my front yard, one of the boys that I went to school with, who was a year ahead of me, came by and made the comment, "You ain't got no breast." First of all, I was shocked that he would say something like that, and second I had no idea he was even looking. I was so embarrassed because other kids were around and heard what he said. I acted like it didn't bother me, but I wanted to run and hide and never show my face again. I became very self-conscious about how my body looked. I stopped wearing clothes that accentuated my body, and if I had to, I would wear a jacket or sweater to cover up.

It didn't matter how often I was told that I was beautiful, I never believed it. I would always find flaws and point them out. Being called ugly as a child did not help with my self-esteem or self-worth. I was teased a lot as a child about my five-finger forehead and my big eyes. Although some of it was done in jest, it planted a seed in my head that something was wrong with the way I looked. To this day, I always want to cover my forehead. Over time I came to love my big beautiful eyes; they are just the right shape for my beautiful face.

That comparison trap carried on into adulthood. I used to try to force myself to love how I looked, but it did not work. I wanted curves, but that's not how my body is shaped. I continually compare myself to others or the world's standard of how women should look. I compared myself to other women so much that I stopped liking the way I looked all together. I didn't even want to look in the mirror because I didn't like what I saw. I used to bite my nails as a child, so I didn't particularly like my hands, and my feet are a whole other story. I often said I didn't care what people thought of me, but the truth is, I did. My self-image was not good at all. I would tell myself the lie; I don't need to lose weight, I look all right just the way I am, knowing I was not content with my weight. Initially, it was because of the images I saw all over the place, but later it was for health reasons. I hardly ever wore makeup, but I started trying to put makeup on. I watched youtube videos and studied how other women applied their makeup, all because I was trying to force myself to feel good about me. But I still would find all kinds of flaws and would often point them out.

I wrote a song about self-image called "Real Beauty." The hook to the song says "Real beauty, where does it come, real beauty, how can I get some, real beauty where does it come from, real beauty how can I get some." The first verse talks about being created in the image of God. The second verse talks about what American society expects us to look like. We buy into the lie that beauty is external, so we do everything to dress up the outer man while neglecting our inner man. God does not look at the outward appearance he looks at the heart. *But the Lord said to Samuel, "Don't judge by his appearance or height, for I have rejected him. The Lord doesn't see things the way you see them. People judge by outward appearance, but the Lord looks at the heart." (I Samuel 16:7 NLT)*

I never even considered that I was made in the image of God, and everything He creates is good. So essentially I was telling myself God made something bad, and that was me. While reading a daily devotional written by Sarah Young, I ran across this statement, "Above all, stop comparing yourself with other people." It went on to say; comparison is wrong and meaningless. Comparing leads to pride or inferiority or both. Stop judging and evaluating yourself because it's not your role to do so.

It took many years before I was able to see the beautiful woman God created. I literally had to tell myself; I am beautiful. I am fearfully and wonderfully made just about every day until I started believing it. God reminded me every time I looked in the mirror that He did not make a mistake when He made me. It took me 52 years to finally realize that I am God's masterpiece. *For we are God's masterpiece. He has created us anew in Christ Jesus, so we can do the good things He has planned for us long ago. (Eph. 2:10 NLT)*

There will always be somebody richer, smarter, or prettier; I just have to keep reminding myself there is no win in comparison. *A peaceful heart leads to a healthy body; jealously is like cancer in the bones. (Proverbs 14:30 NLT)*

I never thought of comparison as jealousy, but actually, it is. You want what someone else has, whether it's their gift, talent, style or calling.

Are you measuring yourself outside of the standard of God, which is Jesus? I was listening to a message by Lisa

Bevere, and she stated in the sermon, "Comparison will rob you of joy." She also asked this question, how have you labeled yourself? Then went on to say we have to strip off those labels we've put on ourselves and see ourselves the way God sees us. I thank God for the men and women going forth and pouring into the masses in this season. Even while watching that sermon, I had to be reminded; I am not too old, my time is coming, God is birthing something out of me. God made me uniquely, and there are people that only I can reach. The same applies to you. Our sisters and brothers are not our competition. There is room for everyone. Ask God what His purpose is for you and ask Him to give you the grace to walk it out and fulfill the destiny He has for you.

Years ago, there was a particular artist that came to town to do a workshop. At no point did I seek to introduce myself to them personally or give them my information. My role was to pick them up and drop them off. After the artist left Peoria, at one of our rehearsals a member of the choir stated, they humbly introduced their self to the artist and gave them their information. I saw this person totally different and humble was not the way I saw them. I saw them as arrogant and self-absorbed. I totally judged them, not out loud but in my heart. I did not know the person's heart or motive. What I saw as arrogance could've just been confidence. Whenever someone compliments me, I humbly defer the gratitude to God, but in this case, I judged them for doing the same thing. They were totally grateful to God for allowing them to even be in the presence of the artist. I had to take a hard look at myself and try to figure out why I judged this person so harshly.

I had an encounter with a recording artist a few years back that wasn't very pleasant. Some friends and I were at a discussion panel session in Vegas, and this artist was one of the panelists. After the panel discussion was over, we were allowed to take pictures with the artists. My friend wanted to take a picture with the artist, so I was trying to get their attention. When the artist finally acknowledged me, they were not pleased that I interrupted their conversation so they approached me with an attitude and stuck out their hand so I could shake it. I shook their hand out of politeness, but I was not the one that wanted a picture with them. I am not starstruck, they are people just like we are. That artist's reaction is why I will not approach an artist. Another reason is I am not bold enough to do what my friend did for fear of being ignored or turned away. Which actually happened.

Theatre will give you a hard lesson in humility. Even though it takes more than one person to have a successful show, people will still come to see one or two people and will sometimes disregard you altogether. That's a hard pill to swallow, but it's true. I was new to the theatre world, so I thought because I had a lead role when the show was over, people would want to greet me as well as the person they came to see. I learned quickly that that wasn't true.

I am very grateful that God chooses to use me the way He does, but I have to remember, that comparison is a trap, don't get entangled in the lie. God made us all unique. To become the woman who God intended me to be, I had to be willing to face myself.

CHAPTER 7

Insignificance

Went to a Homegoing service of a fellow classmate. Usually, friends, family, and others share beautiful stories about the dearly departed. They may also share some funny or not so amusing anecdotes as well. If you did not know that person, you get a glimpse of who they were that day. Their real truth is revealed. After hearing the stories, you may say, I wish I got to know them or I'm glad I didn't experience that side of them. Either way, now that they are no longer here, you will never get to experience them the way those that really knew them did. Several classmates attended the service. It was a bittersweet reunion of sorts. The classmate had not been able to come to other class reunions but was able to participate in what would be their last reunion. I was told this particular classmate would be attending but for the life of me, could not recall who they were. I'm not good at remembering names, but I rarely forget a face.

The minute I saw them, I recognized them immediately. My memory of the classmate is they were always engaged in conversation. Thinking back, I kind of saw them in a parent role when engaged in these conversations. From the stories shared at the service, that classmate was a fantastic parent.

As I stated earlier, the Homegoing service was bittersweet in several ways for me. The day was not about me, and I don't want to seem selfish; however, another part of me that needs to be dealt with reared its ugly head that day. It has shown up before, but I either missed it, dismissed it, or masked it. This day, I tried to conceal it, but it wouldn't let me. That thing that was buried so deep inside me is insignificance.

Google Dictionary's definition of insignificance is the "quality" of being too small or unimportant to be worth consideration.

I was wondering how insignificance could be quality. Then I read Part A of the definition.

Google Dictionary's definition of quality is the standard of something as measured against other things of a similar kind.

I knew the gist of what insignificance meant but seeing it in writing jolted my heart. Then seeing the definition of quality opened my eyes completely to how I labeled myself years ago without realizing it. Because we moved, I had to transfer to another school to start my junior year in high school. The school I transferred from was actually the rival of the school I was transferring to. I was told all sorts of stories about the school I was transferring to, so I had preconceived notions about the school before I even start attending the school. To my surprise, the students at the school I transferred to were more welcoming and much more courteous than the students at my former school. At my former school, I experienced bullying, was degraded and shunned. Except for the people I went to grade school with, not very many people talked to me.

I attended the service with my best friend who I had known since grade school. After the Homegoing service was over, we started greeting our classmates. I figured hardly anyone would remember me so my guard was up and I had already formed a response in my brain, my mask statement. "Nobody remembers me." That's the way I respond when people say they don't remember me. When my best friend mentioned me to a classmate she was greeting, they looked a little puzzled, so I immediately used my mask statement "Nobody remembers me," to which they responded, "Nope I don't remember you" while leaning in to hug me. I replied, "Yes, I was in your class too," as if to subliminally say, Ok, you don't remember me from back then, but we can acknowledge each other next time. I knew who they were and even remembered their name. That classmate was an athlete and a pretty popular one, so they were memorable. There was no more conversation between us, and I was cool with that, or so I thought.

That particular incident reminded me of the label I placed on myself years ago. I did not give it a name back then but as I stated earlier, the ugly label of insignificance reared its ugly head again. After mulling the events of the day over and over again and because I know I'm on this journey to wholeness, I knew this thing had to be uprooted and destroyed. So I asked God to reveal to me the root cause of this thing and where it came from. I did not get an immediate response, but early the Saturday morning after the service He revealed the answer to me. You will recall the story I shared in a previous chapter about being disregarded as a child. The events of that day affected me in more ways than I thought. Being disregarded allowed insignificance to creep in, which caused me to believe I did not matter, and nobody cared. This is the lie that came with being disregarded. I was at all of the required practices to be able to march in the Santa Claus parade but was told I wasn't and still wasn't chosen. What I didn't mention early was the leader who required us to be at all the practices was not at any of them so he could not have known who was there.

I had several encounters throughout childhood and adulthood, where I was fed the lie that I was insignificant, and nobody cared.

I like watching the sitcom King of Queens. On the show Baseball, Doug had to give Arthur, his father-n-law who lives with him, a ride home from work. Arthur talks a lot and sometimes rambles on and on about nothing. On this show, as they were riding home, Arthur was talking non-stop all the way to Queens, which took about an hour and a half. When they arrived home, Arthur told Doug he would make sure he got the book as promised. Doug made Arthur think he was enjoying their conversation and was excited about getting the book and even lied and said he couldn't wait to get it. As soon as Carrie, Doug's wife came home; it was a different story. He told Carrie how Arthur went on and on and how he sounded like an old demented circus monkey. Doug was in the living room. Carrie was in the kitchen. While telling Carrie about his ride home with Arthur, Doug didn't know Carrie went to the garage to get a beer. When Doug walked into the kitchen, Arthur was standing there. Doug wasn't sure Arthur heard what he said about him, so he and Carrie did a reenactment with Carrie in the kitchen acting like her father and Doug in living room repeating what he said about Arthur. Arthur walked into the kitchen during the reenactment and is hurt by what he sees. To make a long story short, Doug and Carrie treat Arthur to a baseball game to try to make amends. They both do something stupid and end up in Mets jail. After the game is over, Arthur, the person they both hurt, was the one who reclaimed them from Mets jail. Be careful how you treat people. The person you disregard may be the one who has to save you.

One of my uncles, I'll call him Jackson, who lived out of town, came to visit. I was at another uncle's house, who I'll call Vincent when my uncle Jackson arrived. I stuck around because I didn't get to see uncle Jackson often and wanted to see him. Uncle Jackson had seen me several times before when he would come to visit. My immediate family, my father, and a few other family members traveled to and attended a birthday celebration for uncle Jackson at his house.

I greeted uncle Jackson with excitement like I always did when he came to town, and I was able to see him. I told him who I was and who I belonged to because he had a puzzled look on his face. His exact words to me were "I thought Lenill (my daddy) only had boys." This wasn't the first time Uncle Jackson said those words to me. He said the same exact words when I was a little girl. Now I was the one with the puzzled look on my face. I stood there for a minute, just as I did as a little girl waiting for an acknowledgment. He didn't really say much else; he just looked at me. The lie of insignificance repeated to me just as it did when I was a little girl; I'm not important enough to be worth consideration.

The lie of insignificance brought along with it low self-esteem, low-self worth, feelings of rejection, depression, suicidal thoughts, and thoughts of worthlessness. Now that I know the root cause of the lie of insignificance, I can begin the healing process, which won't be easy but worth it. In my heart, I already know I am worthy and worth it because Christ gave His life for this messed up, flawed little girl. Now I've got to accept that truth, encourage myself daily, and live like the Daddy's girl that I am. *But you are not like that, for you are a chosen people. You are royal priests, a holy nation, God's very own possession. As a result, you can show others the goodness of God, for he called you out of the darkness into his wonderful light. (1 Peter 2:9 NLT)*

I started this chapter with a classmate's Homegoing service, so I'll end it with this. Although some of my classmates didn't remember me, the classmate's service I attended did remember me. That's the first thing they said to me when we saw each other at the reunion. We sat together and talked just like the classmate used to do with so many others many years ago, not knowing that would be our first and last conversation. I will cherish that memory forever.

CHAPTER 8

Spirit of Unworthiness

I was listening to the sermon The Year of Perspective by Pastor Toure' Roberts of Potter's House One Church Los Angeles. He stated in the message that some people would try to pitch their perspective on you to see if you will answer. He said this because someone from his past called him by his street name back in the day.

What do you answer to? Do you respond to your past hurt, rejection, guilt, or disappointment? Do you answer to distrust, molestation, physical, sexual or mental abuse, or rape? What do you answer to? Sadly, the truth is, I answered to all of my past hurts, but the one thing I answered to loudly is the Spirit of Unworthiness.

You see, that one occurrence of being disregarded also made me feel I was not good enough or worthy enough. From that day on, I always doubted myself. If I were looked over or not chosen for something, I would tell myself it was because I wasn't good enough. Even if I was selected, most times, I felt I did not deserve to be chosen or had to live up to someone else's standards.

I made the cheerleading team when I was in the sixth grade. I was so excited, I ran home and told my step-mother. She was happy for me too. I was very athletic as a child and cheerleading on one of the sports I loved. I adore Track-n-Field. I actually wanted to run in the Olympics one day. I'll speak more on that later, back to cheerleading.

I made the team again my seventh-grade year. I went home and told my step-mother, who didn't say much. That year one of my best friends made the team too. We were so happy to get to do a sport together. Most of the basketball games were on Saturdays. That year we had a bad snowstorm, and an away game, meaning the game was at a different school. Me and three other cheerleaders made it to the game. We did not cheer for the lightweight team, but another cheerleader and I decided to cheer for the heavyweights. The other two cheerleaders refused to participate. Because of their refusal, they got kicked off the team, so there was another tryout. Another one of my best friends made the team in the second tryouts. All was right with the world that year. My best friends and I were cheering together. We had so much fun.

We all made the team our eighth-grade year as well. Of course, we were ecstatic; we got to do it all over again, together. I walked home excited to tell my step-mother the great news. When I entered the house, she was in the kitchen cooking. I walked in the kitchen, still excited but a little apprehensive. "Mom I made the cheerleading team again." She kept cooking, never looked at me, and said: "Why don't they give somebody else a chance?" I walked out of the kitchen in silence and did what I usually did, hid my pain, and acted as if what she said did not phase me, but it actually did. I was hurt because all I ever wanted to do was make her proud. Even though I was chosen, I no longer felt worthy enough to be on the team. I didn't quit, though because I loved cheering. I wanted to cheer in high school too, but I talked myself out of trying out because I didn't know how to do gymnastics. Not knowing intimidated me, so I told myself I was burnt out, but in reality, I never thought I would make the team. I transferred schools after my sophomore year because we moved. My senior year, the cheerleaders had already been chosen, but for some reason, they had a second tryout. I was excited, but again, I talked myself out of trying out because I was intimidated by the gymnastics. I commend those who made an effort to try out whether they could do gymnastics or not. I kicked myself for not even making an effort. I assume gymnastics was not a factor in making the team because not much was used. Unworthiness breeds self-sabotage.

When I was a freshman in high school, I tried out for the track team and made it.

We used to run the halls and stairs, and I absolutely loved it. Well, with my father being the Pastor of the church I attended, I was expected to participate in Sunday School, Bible Study, Prayer Meeting, BYF (Baptist Youth Fellowship) and choir rehearsal. We were allowed to participate in extra-curricular activities, but the church came first. One particular Sunday during the Sunday School hour, it was time to elect Sunday School officers. My father chose me to be the Sunday School secretary. I was 14-years-old at the time. When he told me that's what I was going to do, my response was, "I don't want to. " I don't know if this embarrassed my Dad or not but when we got home, he told me since I didn't want to be the Sunday School secretary, I couldn't run track, so I had to quit the team. Now what one had to do with the other, I'll never know.

I love track and field. That is one sport that I could watch all day long and never get bored. When it was time to try out my sophomore year, because I did not want to put in the work, I used the Sunday School secretary punishment as an excuse. It was true my freshman year, but my Dad had not said anything regarding participating in the sport during my sophomore year. Because I wasn't allowed to run my freshman year, my passion for running began to fade, and my heart wasn't in it anymore. I did run track my junior year, and it felt great. I opted out of running track my senior year. All I wanted to do was graduate and move out of the house. I would have loved to have my parent's support in everything I did, but it wasn't there.

My parents lack of support was disheartening and painful, but I stuffed all of that pain deep inside my vault and acted as if nothing phased me. I learned to stuff my feelings as a child. As the mantra goes, never let them see you sweat; well my mantra was never let them see me cry. If I let anyone see me shed a tear, that would mean I let them get to me. I was never going to give them that satisfaction. But years later, that pain would surface and begin to leak out without me even knowing it was happening.

Unworthiness surfaced in my relationship with my stepmother in a way that affected how I viewed her and how I allowed her to love me. I didn't believe I deserved another mother. I always felt like I was taking her away from her biological children. Instead of dividing her time between six children, it was now divided between 13 children. Even writing this is causing tears to flow because, for some reason, I felt my chance at having a mother ended when I was 3 three years old. Somehow I made up in my mind that my chance at having a mommy ended when mine died. Although my step-mother said she loved me, I didn't believe I was worthy to receive her love. How could she really love children that she didn't carry in her womb and give birth to? My step-mother told me she loved me and even showed me affection, but I realize now I never felt worthy of her love because she did not give birth to me. That's why, as a child, I tried to buy her love with perfection. I tried to be the perfect daughter for her, but I failed over and over again. I could never achieve being perfect because I was born a flawed human being.

One day I was watching The Amazing Dr. Pol. He is a veterinarian who has a reality show. On one of the shows, a young lady brought in some chicks who were lethargic and wouldn't eat. She referred to those chicks as her family. There was also a young woman who lost her pet. I couldn't understand why she was taking it so hard. It was a pet, not a person. Then I had a conversation with a family member who told me if they lost their pet, it would be hard for them as well. If people can see pets as family, why couldn't I understand that my step-mother saw me as one of her children?

Upon reflection, my grandmother passed away after giving birth to my biological mother. My biological mother was raised by her step-mother and step-father. I didn't get to know either of her step-parents well, but I did get to meet her step-father, and I believe their love for my biological mother was genuine, and they viewed her as their own child. I now understand that me thinking I was unworthy of my step-mother's love was my perception and not necessarily true.

CHAPTER 9

The Search for Significance

In her experience, "All girls marry their fathers." Iyanla Vanzant.

Even though I watched this particular episode before, when I heard her say those words this time, it resonated in my spirit. I had a conversation with God two days earlier about that very statement.

My Dad was a hard worker and a great provider. Although he lived in the home, he was always gone. He was a Pastor, so he was gone continuously doing church stuff. The times he was in the house, he was not there emotionally. I remember a time one of my friends and I went to a service at the church where my father was the Pastor. I left the church many years before, but would still go back and visit. As soon as he saw her, he greeted her with excitement and hugged her really tight. My Dad was not the kind of person who showed us a lot of affection, so I was totally shocked and hurt by what I witnessed. He also was not big on saying I love you; he would say it in the form of a question, "You know I love you, right?"

As a child, I always wanted to jump in my Daddy's lap and hug him tight around the neck and him hug me back. That didn't happen, but we did have a bedtime ritual, I would kiss him on the cheek every night before I went to bed. The kiss on the cheek was my way of saying, "I love you, goodnight." Even when I kissed him on the cheek, he would sit there like a stone and showed no emotion. I didn't care at the time. He was my Daddy, and I loved him.

One night when I was about nine or ten years old, I went to kiss him goodnight, but he moved away from me. I left his room confused because he had never done that before. His actions that night ended our bedtime ritual and me showing that kind of affection to my father. I always felt like I was kept at arm's length. I would have been satisfied just laying my head on his shoulder or even touching elbows, but I felt I did not have permission to do so. He reached for and held my hand one time that I remember, as an adult. I was shocked, but it felt right. I will cherish that memory forever.

Reflecting on my childhood, most girls want boys to like them even though most of the time, all they wanted to do was feel you up. I had that experience several times, I was naïve in thinking they actually liked me, but when they were done, they moved on to the next girl. One day my sister and I were out walking, and we saw a group of boys. One of them wanted to talk to my sister. We both walked over to the boys; there were about three or four of them. Not one of them even looked my way or said hello. I stood there awkwardly while all of them tried to hit on my sister. Although I longed for attention, the little I got was usually not what I wanted. As an adult, one of my guy friends told me the reason guys didn't hit on me is they knew I wouldn't bite. They would usually go for easy girls. Now let me clarify, I am definitely not saying my sister was easy, that couldn't be farther from the truth. My sister is very confident in herself, and she carries herself that way. I was not as confident, and it showed. I didn't think much of myself, so I assumed no one else did either. What brews on the inside will undoubtedly find a way to surface and leak out.

> "We attract what we are, not what we want."
> **Kimberly Jones-Pothier**

As an adult, I still received unwanted attention from men. I often wondered what they saw when they looked at me. Did I send them the wrong message? Did they take my kindness for something else? I am not flirtatious, don't even know how to be, but it seemed I kept sending the wrong signal to men. I started telling myself that men only wanted me for what they thought they could get from me, my body. So I put on the "don't approach me mask" whenever I'm around men. They see it as me looking mean, but I'm not a mean person. I just want them to see past my the exterior and see my heart. I am more than just my body.

I was very fortunate to marry a hard-working man who is a great provider, just like my father. He takes good care of his family. He is also kind and patient like my father and always willing to lend a helping hand. We've had several bumps and bruises along the way in our many years together, and by the grace of God we made it through and learned from the mistakes, but the emotional part of our union is suffocating. I love him deeply; however, what I need from him is intimacy. That is one of the things that is missing in our marriage.

I over-love my children and under-love my husband. By that, I mean, I am open with my children and made it very comfortable for them to share everything with me. I made a vow that when I had children, I was going to make sure they knew I loved them and that they could come to me whenever they needed to with no judgment. I did not have that with either of my parents. When it comes to my husband, I'm not as open with him. Because of the dynamic of our relationship, it's not that easy to open up to him. Part of that is due to the lack of trust that I carried over from my previous relationship. Like my father, he does not show a lot of emotion, so sometimes I don't feel safe sharing things with him. However, my husband is the one person I should be able to be completely open with.

When God called me to preach I was hesitant about telling my husband. I was afraid of what his reaction may be. It took me a few weeks before I felt brave enough to tell him. To my surprise, he was totally supportive and encouraging.

God knew I would need my husband's support and encouragement because I was in a very broken state. I had been unfaithful in my marriage. I knew it was wrong, but I did it anyway. Thank our Heavenly Father for forgiveness. I was searching for something no one could give me, and that was love and significance. I love deeply, and once I let you in my heart, I usually don't let go. The same love I gave is the same love I wanted from others. I wanted to be somebody's number one. I wanted to matter. I placed high expectations on others that I couldn't even fulfill myself. I didn't love myself enough to matter to me. My husband told me one day; I won't let anybody love me. I didn't understand what he meant at the time but looking back; he was right. I had been hurt so many times in life that I started closing my heart to be able to receive love, even from myself.

I had only been in two real relationships, and because I was hurt in the first relationship, it warped my view of any other relationship I would have in the future. I did not allow myself to heal before entering the next relationship. I viewed all men the same; I didn't think any of them were capable of being faithful. I brought a lot of baggage into my current relationship, lack of trust, low self-worth, low self-esteem, and my guard was always up. I was not going to let anybody hurt me again, so I wouldn't give myself completely to anyone. I gave myself entirely in my first relationship and was taken for granted, so I was not letting that happen again. Unfortunately, me trying to protect myself from getting hurt again affected my marriage. I am grateful that my husband didn't throw in the towel and end our marriage. He was and is very patient with me.

It wasn't until I was in my 50s that I even thought about who I am in Christ. I wore so many masks that I completely lost my real identity. As a child, up to the age of six years old, I remember being bold, unashamed, fearless, free, and happy. After my father remarried, life changed for me. I became reserved, bashful, reticent, and subdued. Because I do not like confusion, I would sometimes go along just to get along. There were also times I would say and do things I did not want to do to keep the peace. Because I went along to get along so much, people thought they could take advantage of me, and sometimes I let them. I was labeled with things that were not true like I was a pushover, rude, mean, nosey, and a miss know-it-all. I began to believe those things about me, which made me dislike myself even more. I became a loner anxiously waiting to escape childhood.

To quote lyrics from Whitney Houston's "Greatest Love of All," the greatest love of all is easy to achieve. Learning to love yourself it is the greatest love of all. I am still learning to love who I am. The woman who God designed me to be. God is love. How can I not adore what the creator of love created?

My beloved friends, let us continue to love each other since love comes from God. Everyone who loves is born of God and experiences a relationship with God. The person who refuses to love doesn't know the first thing about God, because God is love-so you can't know Him if you don't love. This is how God showed His love for us: God sent His only son into the world so we might live through Him. This is the kind of love we are talking about not that we were once upon a time loved by God, but that He loved us and sent His son as a sacrifice to clear away our sins and the damage they've done to our relationship with God. (1 John 4:7 -10 MSG)

I was so blinded by self-hatred that I couldn't love myself. I could sincerely lavish love on everybody else but couldn't bring myself to love me. Until I learned to love myself, I would always be searching for love and significance. It would take years for me to find the strength to finally love me.

CHAPTER 10

Who Does Your Influence Come From

Where does your influence come from? Your mother, father, a family friend, teacher, or mentor? Sometimes we hear the words "you act just like your mother or you're just like your father." In some instances that may be true. Our influence comes from the people we grow up with it or a favorite teacher or mentor. I did not grow up with my biological mother; everything I learned about womanhood came from my step-mother. Although I have a lot of my father's traits, she is the parent who influenced me the most.

When I first moved out on my own, I didn't know a lot about life. I was nineteen years old with a seven-month-old son I was responsible for. I made a lot of mistakes with him. He was my firstborn. Being that I had never been a mother before I leaned on my step-mother a lot. She used to tell me do not talk baby gibberish to him, talk to him just like I spoke to her. I listened but still was unsure about a lot of things. I did learn that for your baby to learn how to talk; you actually have to show them how by talking to them. Don't judge me; I was young, I didn't know.

I used to watch how my Dad took care of the house. He made sure all the bills were paid, and we never went hungry. If we did, it was by our choice. To this day, I make sure all of my bills are paid and paid on time. It's an excellent practice. Believe it or not, paying your bills late, also affects your credit. He also had a great work ethic. He worked hard until the day he was laid off. He then became a full-time Pastor. He worked equally as hard as a Pastor, which was great for the church but not for his family. He spent more time at the church than he did with us. He was old school; the church came first. I found myself putting ministry before family as well. It was what was modeled in front of me, so that is what I thought we were supposed to do. Me putting ministry first became a problem in my marriage. Just like my father, I spent a lot of time at the church several days a week and hardly any time with my family. When I learned better, I did better. The role should be God, family, church. God created family years before the "church," for lack of a better word, was established.

I watched how my step-mother took care of the household. My step-mother cooked and cleaned and took care of all thirteen of us children plus my father. I find myself doing some of the things I learned from her in regards to cooking and cleaning. She would often get on my case about the way I sat. I was a tomboy growing up so sometimes I would sit like a guy with my legs open. It was comfortable for me. She would always remind me to close my legs and sit like a lady. We were also not allowed to slouch. She told us to sit up straight, which promoted good posture. To this day, I do not slump. I did not like to carry a purse either; she was ok with that. Once I had a child, she told me I needed to start carrying one, so I did. It took some getting used to, but I finally got the hang of it. These are just a few things I learned growing up. My step-mother also, along with being a wife and mother, was a Sunday School and BYF teacher, youth choir president, church musician, and First Lady. It was only by the grace of God that she was able to wear so many hats. Watching her wear all of those hats, which was not easy, taught me how to multi-task and persevere. I commend her greatly. She had a significant influence on the youth of the church. To this day, they still mention how wonderful she was.

My oldest granddaughter is learning how to drive. Her father, our oldest son, gave her the task to find the route between her home and place of worship. He gave her a map, the name of the street she lives on and the name of the street where she worships. He gave her a starting and ending point. She was to find the route between. My husband reminded me that whenever we traveled out of town, he would have our son read the map. Now you may say like father like son. Well, my husband is not our son's biological father, but our son is so much like him because that's where his influence came from. I see so much of my husband in both of our sons. From the way they talk to how they run their households. My husband often jokes that he is a lot like his father as well. I also am like my father in a lot of ways. I do some of the things he used to do and say some things he used to say. Some of our mannerisms come from our parents too. They are deep-rooted. Our parents, our biggest influencers, were our role models.

Others influence us as well. As a child, I looked up to a lot of people and wanted to be like a few of them. There was one particular person I watched all of the time. I watched how they carried themselves and their overall interaction with people. I also observed their walk with the Lord. This person was not married, but kept having children, which meant they were having sex, but there were no consequences. Because I knew that person was a believer, I figured it must be ok to have sex before marriage, and if you happen to get pregnant, there would be no consequences. The more I studied and grew spiritually, the more I learned, and that was not true. We have to be careful about how we live our lives before others because you never know who is watching. *Let no one despise you for your youth, but set the believers an example in speech, in conduct, in love, in faith, in purity (I Timothy 4:12 ESV)*

Who do you pattern your life after? The older I get, the more I want to please God. Our most significant example of how to live life is Jesus Christ. Just as He was in this world but not of this world, so are we. We are citizens of the Kingdom so we should strive to be more like Christ. We are ambassadors of Christ and want to represent Him well. I know there are a lot of outside influences in our lives that shape the way we think and act; however, we have Jesus as our perfect example, we have the Holy Spirit to guide us, and we have the Word of God to direct us. *You are the salt of the earth, but if salt has lost its taste, how shall its saltiness be restored? It is no longer good for anything except to be thrown out and trampled under people's feet. You are the light of the world. A city set on a hill cannot be hidden. Nor do people light a lamp and put it under a basket, but on a stand, and it gives light to all in the house. In the same way, let your light shine before others, so that they may see your good works and give glory to your Father who is in heaven. (Matthew 5:13-16 ESV)*

Our parents meant well, but they could only model for us what they learned from their parents and others who influenced them. The Bible is a great guide to show us how to treat others and live and love like Christ. My only regret is that I did not start studying the Bible when I was younger. I learned from Sunday School lessons and BYF lessons, but I did not read on my own. I pretty much held onto my father's coat tail until I moved out on my own and changed churches. It was then that I started learning how to study God's word for myself.

CHAPTER 11

The Girl Behind the Veil

I mentioned earlier in this book that my biological mother's death made me feel as if she abandoned me. I don't believe it was intentional, but from what I was told, she had uncontrolled high blood pressure and was in the hospital a lot. I also do not know what caused her uncontrolled blood pressure, but what I do know is it was so high it caused her to have a stroke and die. I'm not blaming her for passing away, but she did, and we were left without a mother.

Holding on to stagnant pain will stunt your growth. It's called arrested development. Iyanla Vanzant.

I forgive you, mommy, for leaving me. I have to grow up the little girl in me that is still yearning for her mommy who wasn't there.

While doing some research about girls losing their mother at an early age, I ran across a blog titled 17 Things Girls Need from their Mothers, author unknown. Some of the things listed are:

- **To be told she's beautiful** – Not because of what she is wearing, you definitely can complement her on that, but she needs to know her beauty comes from within. *Your beauty should not come from outward adornments, such as elaborate hairstyles and the wearing of gold jewelry or fine clothes. Rather, it should be that of your inner self, the unfading beauty of a gentle and quiet spirit, which is of great worth in God's sight. (1 Peter 3:3-4 NIV)*

- **To know her self-worth** – She needs to know her worth is not in her body. She is a rare jewel. She is so much more than her shape. *She is more precious than rubies; nothing you desire can compare with her. Long life is in her right hand; in her left hand are riches and honor. Her ways are pleasant ways, and all her paths are peace. She is a tree of life to those who take hold of her; those who hold her fast will be blessed. (Proverbs 3:15-18 NIV)*

- **To be shown how to love** – She needs to know how to love herself first, then her husband and her children. Show her by example, what unconditional love looks like. *For God so loved the world, that He gave His only begotten Son, that whosoever believeth in Him should not perish, but have everlasting life (John 3:16 KJV)*

- **To be gentle and strong** – She needs to know how to be soft, yet firm. She needs to know when to concede and when to stand her ground. *For God has not given us a spirit of fear and timidity, but of power, love, and self-discipline. (2 Timothy 1:7 MSG)*

- **To know who she is** – She needs to know her likes and dislikes. She needs to know that she does not have to go along with the crowd, she can be her own person. She needs to form her own identity, have a sense of self and love who she is. *For we are God's masterpiece. He has created us anew in Christ Jesus, so we can do the good things he planned for us long ago. (Ephesians 2:10 NLT)*

- **To see her mother love her father** – She needs to know what real love looks like. *And further, submit to one another out of reverence for Christ. For wives, this means submit to your husbands as to the Lord. For husbands, this means love your wives, just as Christ loved the church. He gave up His life for her to make her holy and clean, washed by the cleansing of God's word. (Ephesians 5:21-22, 25-26 NLT)*

- **To talk about sex** – She needs to know that she can come to you and talk freely about sex. She needs to understand that it's more than just a physical act. Her heart and emotions are involved, as well. She also needs to know and understand that her body is not to be given to just anybody. *Do you not know that your bodies are temples of the Holy Spirit, who is in you, whom you have received from God? You are not your own; you were bought with a price. Therefore, honor God with your bodies. (1 Corinthians 6:19-20 ESV)*

- **To believe in and be herself** – She needs to believe she is worthy, she is worth it and can accomplish anything she puts her mind to. She needs to be allowed the space to find who she is, whether quiet and reserved or loud and outgoing. Allow her to find herself and celebrate who she is. *You saw me before I was born. Every day of my life was recorded in your book. Every moment was laid out before a single day had passed. How precious are* *your thoughts about me, O God. They cannot be numbered! (Psalm 139:16-17 NLT)*

- **To respect** – She needs to be taught how to respect herself first, then how to respect others. *Do to others whatever you would like them to do to you. This is the essence of all that is taught in the law and the prophets. (Matthew 7:12 NLT)*

- **To know she is loved** – She needs to know you love her unconditionally even when you feel she does not love you. Be there for her in good times and not so good times. She needs to know you have her back no matter what. Even if she makes mistakes, which she will, she needs to know you won't disown, degrade or leave her. *Love is patient, love is kind. It does not envy, it does not boast, it is not proud. It does not dishonor others, it is not self-seeking, it is not easily angered, it keeps no record of wrongs. Love does not delight in evil but rejoices with the truth. It always protects, always trusts, always hopes, always perseveres. (1 Corinthians 13:4- 7 NIV)*

I tailored these things to fit my needs; however, I believe they can benefit everyone.

I used to care what people thought about me even though I said I didn't. I didn't know who I was, so sometimes I would believe what was said about me and start living that way. I wore a lot of masks that did not fit my personality, which caused people to think I was mean, boring, or a pushover, etc. Because I didn't trust people, I would wear my protective mask a lot to try to keep people from hurting me. It worked to a certain extent until I let my guard down a little and let people in. Every time without fail, I would end up getting hurt, so I started trying to close my heart off, but God called me out on that.

I was involved in a youth prison ministry. We made visits to male and female youth prisons. Before we made the visits we would meet together, strategize and pray. At one of the meetings, a team member who has the gift of discernment was asked to pray. I had recently been hurt by a person who was supposed to be my friend. When the team member prayed for me, the Holy Spirit through her, exposed the prayer I had prayed to God about not accepting any more friends in my life. The Holy Spirit also said through her that God did not tell me to close my heart off. Because my private prayer to God had been exposed, I thought God was disappointed with me and depression set in. I couldn't really talk to anyone about it because I didn't know how and no one reached out me. For weeks, I tried to minister in song with the praise team and choir, but I was just going through the motions. My spirit was broken. I was eventually asked not to minister with the praise team, which broke my spirit even more.

After gaining strength to reach out, I was finally able to share what I was dealing with. I was prayed for and encouraged and eventually came out of the depression. I realized that God was not disappointed in me. He loves me no matter what. I also kept my heart open to receive whoever the Lord wanted to bring in my life. What I didn't say earlier is I wore the depression on my face. I couldn't smile or laugh; I could barely function. As I stated above, I was just going through the motions. Because no one reached out to me in my time of need, I try to reach out and connect with others, especially if I can clearly see they are hurting.

I lived my life trying to fit in. All I wanted was to be accepted and validated. But I sought validation in the wrong places. I kept trying to get validation from people who could never approve of me because they did not create me. I accepted the labels people put on me because I thought they could see something in me or about me that I couldn't. Some other labels put on me were quiet and shy, or as stated before, people thought I was a pushover because I didn't say much. I was also given labels like sweet, humble, and kind.

There was a particular situation that happened that caused a lot of confusion and because I stood my ground and didn't back down like they thought I would, I was labeled the devil's daughter by the people I conflicted with. That label hurt me to my core. That was the very first time I experienced church hurt. I never understood what that term meant until I experienced it for myself. We, the church, which is not the building but the people, are supposed to love each other, but instead, we tear each other down, especially if titles are involved. During that time in my life, I discovered some things in me that were not good. I never want anything wrong to happen to people, but I was actually happy when something terrible happened to one of the people I was in conflict with. I had to do some soul searching and repenting. It took me a while to forgive those people, but to be able to move forward, I had to forgive them. Forgiveness is not for the offender; it is for you.

Listening to a message by Pastor Sarah Jakes-Roberts of Potter's House One Church LA, she asked the question, who are you at your core? The most important part of who we are is not what people see or enjoy; it's our core. Most of the time you see my outer shell. Unless you really know me, you never see my essence, my inner being, mainly because of significant trust issues but also because I really didn't know who I was.

Do you know who you are? Do you know how you operate? Do you understand what you operate from? Do you operate from brokenness, anger, low esteem, hurt, pain, disappointment? Most times, we operate from our default setting. That thing that shaped us into who we are. It could be something that happened in your childhood, (e.g., sexual abuse, abandonment, physical or mental abuse, depression, etc.)

What is your go-to when unexpected events throw you off course? Do you snap out or fall silent, fight or flight? Because I have to control everything I can in my life, I immediately start fussing and complaining, whether valid or not, or I shut down totally and distance myself from the situation. I also ponder on and overthink things which causes me to second guess and doubt.

To discover your true identity, the fact of being who or what a person or thing is, ask God. You can simply say, Lord, who am I? Earnestly seek Him, He will show you. Get in alignment, a position or agreement or alliance with God. Ask Him to show you who He created you to be, then allow Him to strip away that outer shell, that default setting, so you can begin your path to healing. *Search me, O God, and know my heart; test me and know my anxious thoughts. Point out anything in me that offends You, and lead me along the path of everlasting life. Psalms 139:23-24 NLT)*

Once you discover and start walking in the new you, you're going to have to learn how to navigate in and protect the new you. Be careful not to fall back to the person you used be, navigating out of brokenness. Always seek to operate in the new you. Make decisions from the person you are now. But, get ready for the battle within, because the old you will fight not to lose its identity to the new you. The former you will continuously struggle to control you and can sabotage your destiny. Allow yourself the space to make mistakes but be careful not to fall back into the old you. We have to die to ourselves daily to become who God created us to be. Pray that God will change you from the inside out and trust that He will.

While reading the book Wholeness, God started showing me what I was operating from, Fallacy of Perfection, Disregard, Rejection, Spirit of Comparison, Insignificance, Search for Significance, Girl Behind the Veil who was bullied, shunned, molested, rejected, put down and who experienced church hurt, in order to get me ready for purpose. He is still revealing daily, those broken pieces that shaped my life. I will reiterate, this journey is not easy, and it's painful. Sometimes the pain seems unbearable, and it feels like God is nowhere around. It's at those times that we need to trust Him even when we can't trace Him. Where I am in my journey is where God needs me to be so He can teach me.

Today I am thankful for Authenticity! I tried to be the way others said I should be for quite some time. But later discovered you'll never measure up to the expectation of people. I, instead, traded their expectations for my own identity. Feels fantastic to be me, always evolving and yet at my fullest extent. I look forward to my days ahead. I look forward to enjoying life as it comes. I've learned to turn the focus away from my best-supporting actress and extras in my own film. I am the main character. I have a lot of lines, and as long as I stay true to my role, there will always be an audience. Be your own star. Chase after you. There is only one you.

Natasha Poole

Daily yielding my will to God is imperative. *Do not copy the behavior and customs of this world, but let God transform you into a new person by changing the way you think. Then you will learn to know God's will for you, which is good and pleasing and perfect (Romans 12:2 NLT)*

Until we care more about God's will than our will, we will remain the way we are. Transformation cannot take place until we yield our will to His will. If you want to change, seek God's will for your life.

CHAPTER 12

The Wrap Up

Super Bowl Sunday 2019. Wow, what a day. God started downloading in me early in the wee hours of the morning. I learned a whole lot about myself that day. This girl knows she's a work in progress, but I never knew so much was buried so deep inside me. The Lord had to dig deep, break up, and excavate some things I never knew existed.

I've been told by different people that I am strong, confident, the way I enter a room or platform is graceful, poised, you're stoic you have this aura about you. And then other people say you're boring or she's so mean or they say lighten up, don't be so serious. What nobody knew is all those descriptions couldn't be farther from the truth. I learned as a child to hide how I really felt inside. I wouldn't let anybody see me cry, not even my father and stepmother. Even when I got a whipping, I would make the sound like I was sobbing, but I wouldn't let a tear fall. I asked God why I held my tears even though I was hurting? He brought to my memory my father, after punishing me, would tell me to dry up. That meant wipe those tears and be quiet. You have to understand my dad was my world; I didn't want to do anything to disappoint him, so when he told me to do something I did it quickly. In reality, I am such a crybaby. Even though I won't let most people see me cry, I cry a lot. Crying is therapy. You feel so much better after you've had a good cry.

I still didn't quite understand how my father telling me to dry up, affected my life now, so I asked for more clarity. The revelation I received from that memory is because my dad told me to dry up; I wasn't allowed to let myself feel. I couldn't just let my heartbreak or feel the pain of rejection, abandonment, or disappointment. I stuffed those feelings down and put on the mask of strength or confidence, or I put on the mask of protection by appearing to look mean. To be honest, I don't know what that mean face looks like because at times it is mistaken for my concentration face. When I'm really concentrating on something, people always tell me to "smile." I'm not mad; I'm just really focused.

I mentioned in an earlier chapter that there is a mask I wear to keep men away from me. Another one of my protective "false faces." That mask says, "Don't even try it," which again gives the misconception that I'm a mean person. In reality, I genuinely love people. The Lord has filled me with compassion for people. I want to see everybody win. I love to laugh and have fun. I'm very flexible, probably to a fault. I'm a natural encourager. I'm clumsy and a goofball because I don't think we need to be serious all the time. I lack confidence, but God is showing me my confidence in him. One truth I will share about myself that I couldn't clearly see until now is how vain I can be. Not proud to admit it, but it's true. I used to tell my husband he was conceited, not realizing that what I saw in him was in me as well. I had this crazy thought to leave instructions for my children to put gloves on my hands if my nails are jacked up when I pass away. I never told them, but that's one of the thoughts I had rolling around in my head - another way of trying to be perfect, even in death.

One of the reasons I love to act is I get to portray a character. It's a chance to escape reality. For a few months, a few hours a night, I get to be someone else. Truth be told, every character I portrayed had a little bit of me or what I thought was me in it.

I'm so glad God is digging up and excavating all of that stuff out of me. During the excavation, everything won't be neat and clean. It's going to be downright dirty and nasty. God is cleaning us out, and it's not going to be easy. He brings us through situations sometimes unscathed, and sometimes, there are scars. There are times God will bring us out of a crisis only for us to go right back to the same thing we were just delivered from. We often think that God will get us out of that situation the same way He did before. Don't assume you know how God will deliver you because you've been through this or something similar previously. Remember, we are unique. Every situation will not be the same. It may look the same, but it's still unique. You don't know how God works. He is the same and never changes, but that doesn't mean He does things the same way.

Life is a lesson. We have many trials, tests, and storms. While watching the sermon Smashing Mirrors by Pastor Travis Greene of Forward City Church, he made the statement "The whole point of the storm is to see God different. Every part of your story matters, good and bad." We all have a purpose; it's up to us to seek God for it. We may be going in a different direction, but as Pastor Greene also stated, purpose interrupts and redirects your life. The shift is necessary because God is equipping you for what He is calling you to do. He also said you've been living by reality when you are called to live by revelation. Reality is what you see; revelation is what you hear. The Holy Spirit made that last statement real clear to me, and it made so much sense. We walk by faith, not by sight. I recommend you watch the whole sermon. It will give you clarity and revelation.

Sometimes when bad things happen to us, or we receive an unfavorable diagnosis, we start blaming the devil. We need to stop blaming the devil for everything we go through; sometimes God allows our test or trial. We can use the story of Job as an example. If you're not familiar with it, read the book of Job in the Bible. Satan was going back and forth in the earth, seeking someone to devour. God asked him have you tried my servant Job? To make a long story short, Job lost everything, his health was challenged, and his friends accused him of sin, God knew Job was faithful, so he allowed the devil to attack him. The devil is a created being. God created him, and because he wants to be God, he twists the things God allows and makes you think they are bad, but they are really for our good. I know it's hard for us to understand this while we are in the midst of our trial, but we've got to get to the place where we really trust that God is working for our good and His glory. *Dear brothers and sisters, when troubles of any kind come your way, consider it an opportunity for great joy. For you know that when your faith is tested, your endurance has a chance to grow. (James 1:2-3 NLT)*

As I am writing this book, I said to God, "It's a bunch of stories about me, it needs to be deeper." He told me, "Sometimes the stories of others need to be heard." You never know how your story can touch someone else. Tell your story. It may not be in a book, but it may be at a coffee shop, a restaurant, pillow talk, or table time. Share your story; you never know who it may help. My purpose for writing this book is to help others start their journey to wholeness. Here are some steps that helped me begin my journey:

Face Yourself

Not an easy thing to do. I had faced the fact that I am not perfect, and I don't have to be. I also had to recognize my strengths and weaknesses. There are things I'm great at, and there are things I suck at. I can be very friendly, or I will ignore you as if you don't exist. That is my truth. Accept who you are right now and seek change. Know that change is not easy. In fact, it is excruciating at times, but it is essential for growth.

Know Your Triggers

Self-awareness is important. Know what takes you out of pocket, upsets you, or makes you angry. Be mindful of what makes you sad, happy, or fearful. To know your triggers, you must have a sense of self. It took me years to learn my triggers, and I am still learning.

Embrace Who You Are Becoming

I have to continually remind myself I am on a journey to becoming who God created me to be. I am still changing, growing, and evolving. Change involves loss, risk, and energy. You may feel a sense of loss when you step out of your comfort zone, those things that defined you, and start embracing who you are becoming. There is also the risk of trying something new or different. You are used to who you were. You know how to navigate through life as the old you. Learning to navigate through life as the new you will be challenging yet rewarding. And lastly, change involves energy. You have to put in the work to change, evolve, and grow. It is not going to happen overnight. Real change takes time and effort.

Trust the Process

We are God's workmanship. Allow Him to mold you into the amazing, extraordinary, beautiful work of art He intends for you to be. Wholeness is a never-ending process, but the result is phenomenal.

Everything that God made is good. He makes no mistakes. Thank You for making me so wonderfully complex! Your workmanship is marvelous - how well I know it. (Ps. 139:14)

It took me a lot of years to start seeing myself the way God sees me. I would often say I'm a King's Kid or I'm a child of the Most High King, but until I actually believed it in my heart, those were just mere words.

I loved hearing people tell me I look just my mother or your mother was so pretty, you look just like her. Although I believe I look like my mother; I look like my father as well, I never thought I was as pretty as she was. God is very patient with me. Although I walk tall with my head held high, He knew I was battling with low self-esteem and low self-worth, and I'm so glad He didn't give up on me. This journey is just beginning, and I'm in for the long haul.

"Daily growth is the goal. Keeping your life situations understood is the mission. Never make excuses for your past. Learn, build, grow, and keep your haters in your rearview."
Benjamin Lamar Thornton

About the Author

Juanita R. Williams is a native of Peoria, Illinois. She is one of 13 children and the daughter of a Pastor. She is a licensed minister, singer, actress and songwriter. She released an EP "Expected Glory" in 2017. Her passion for God, serving God's people, music, and the arts have ignited a passion that requires Juanita to now share the ministry God has given her through writing. Fulfilling her God-given assignment, she wrote her first book, Finding Purpose After Sexual Abuse and Trauma, Life Beyond Pain and Finding My True Identity in God to bring healing and hope to the broken.

www.ingramcontent.com/pod-product-compliance
Lightning Source LLC
Chambersburg PA
CBHW061504250726
48657CB00005B/1725